Fifth Edition, Revised Reprint

Certified Coding Specialist (CCS) Exam Preparation

Jennifer Hornung Garvin,
PhD, MBA, RHIA, CPHQ, CCS,
CTR, FAHIMA

AHIMA PRESS

ISBN 978-1-58426-419-4
AHIMA Product No. AC400413

AHIMA Staff:
Jessica Block, MA, Assistant Editor
Katherine M. Greenock, MS, Production Development Editor
Jason O. Malley, Director, Creative Content Development
Pamela Woolf, Managing Editor

For more information, including updates, about AHIMA Press publications, visit http://www.ahima.org/publications/updates.aspx

American Health Information Management Association
233 North Michigan Avenue, 21st Floor
Chicago, Illinois 60601-5809
ahima.org

Contents

Online Assessments

Practice Multiple Choice and Multiple Select Questions and Answers
Practice Exam 1 Multiple Choice and Multiple Select Questions and Answers
Practice Exam 2 Multiple Choice and Multiple Select Questions and Answers

About the Author

Jennifer Hornung Garvin, PhD, MBA RHIA, CPHQ, CCS, CTR, FAHIMA is currently a Core Research Investigator at the Salt Lake City VA IDEAS Research Center and an Associate Professor at the University of Utah School of Medicine in the Department of Bioinformatics. She is a health information management (HIM) professional with 29 years of experience in HIM and applied informatics. She received an associate of science and a post-baccalaureate certificate in HIM from Gwynedd-Mercy College, bachelor's and doctoral degrees from Temple University, a master's degree in business (MBA) from St. Joseph's University, and a graduate certificate in biomedical informatics from the Oregon Health and Science University. Her professional training includes a postdoctoral fellowship at the Center for Health Equity Research and Promotion (CHERP) sponsored by the Department of Veteran Affairs (VA) at the Philadelphia VA Medical Center (PVAMC) in association with the University of Pennsylvania School of Medicine (SOM). She is an AHIMA-approved ICD-10-CM/PCS trainer.

She was the program director of AHIMA accredited associate's and bachelor's degree program as well as an AHIMA approved coding certificate at Gwynedd-Mercy College for nine years before seeking research training. Dr. Garvin is currently the president of the Utah Health Information Management Association and served as an elected member of the International Healthcare Terminology Standards Development Organization (IHTSDO) Content Committee for 2 years. She has also served on the AHIMA Board of Directors, as chair of the AHIMA Research Committee, and as president of Pennsylvania Health Information Management Association (PHIMA), and the Lehigh Valley Health Information Management Association (LVHIMA) among other HIM volunteer leadership roles. She champions the need for quality data to improve health and healthcare.

Acknowledgments

The author wishes to thank the following individuals for being editors, reviewers, and publishers of previous editions of the *CCS Exam Success Review Book* and *CCS Exam Preparation:*

Elizabeth Forrestal, PhD, RHIA, CCS, FAHIMA
Kathy Arner, LPN, RHIT, CCS, CPC
Genevive Badroe
Christine Staropoli, MS, RHIA, CCS
Angela Picard Carney, PhD, RHIA
Stephen Weiner, DO
Julian Wade Farrior, PhD
Pam Farrior, RPh
Aileen Stanton, CHCO, CCS, CCP
Pauline Graham, RHIT, CHCO, CCS, CCP
Becky Thorson, RHIT, CCS
Linda Donahue, RHIT, CCS, CCS-P, CPC
Christina Benjamin, MA, RHIA, CCS, CCS–P
Dasantila Sherifi, MBA, RHIA

And any other reviewers from past editions who were inadvertently not named.

In addition, a special thank you goes to all the HIM professionals who have sent me questions and suggestions regarding the contents of this book. You have made this work extra special.

I also so much appreciate the helpful AHIMA publication staff members who have assisted in the production of this text.

About the CCS Exam

Coding professionals who pass the certified coding specialist (CCS) exam are professionals skilled in classifying medical data from patient records, generally in the hospital setting. These coding practitioners review patients' records and assign numeric codes for each diagnosis and procedure. To perform this task, they must possess expertise in the ICD-9-CM and CPT coding systems. In addition, the CCS is knowledgeable of medical terminology, disease processes, and pharmacology. Hospitals or medical providers report coded data to insurance companies, or to the government in the case of Medicare and Medicaid recipients, for reimbursement of expenses. Researchers and public health officials also use coded medical data to monitor patterns and explore new interventions. Coding accuracy is thus highly important to healthcare organizations because of its impact on revenues and describing health outcomes, and in fact, certification is becoming an implicit industry standard. Accordingly, the CCS credential demonstrates tested data quality and integrity skills in a coding practitioner. The CCS certification exam assesses mastery proficiency in coding rather than entry-level skills. Professionals experienced in coding inpatient and outpatient records should consider obtaining this certification. For exam eligibility requirements, visit ahima.org/certification.

The National Commission for Certifying Agencies (NCCA) has granted accreditation to AHIMA's certified coding specialist (CCS) certification program for demonstrating compliance with the NCCA Standards for the Accreditation of Certification Programs. NCCA is the accrediting body of the Institute for Credentialing Excellence (formerly the National Organization for Competency Assurance).

The NCCA Standards were created in 1977 and updated in 2003 to ensure that certification programs adhere to modern standards of practice for the certification industry. AHIMA joins an elite group of more than 100 organizations representing more than 200 programs that have received and maintained NCCA accreditation. More information on the NCCA is available online at http://www.credentialingexcellence.org/ncca.

Exam Competency Statements

The CCS certification exam is based on an explicit set of competencies. These competencies were determined by job analysis surveys of hospital-based coders. The competencies are subdivided into domains and tasks, as listed here. The CCS exam tests only content pertaining to the following competencies.

Domain I: Health Information Documentation (9%)

1. Interpret health record documentation using knowledge of anatomy, physiology, clinical disease processes, pharmacology, and medical terminology to identify codeable diagnoses and/or procedures.
2. Determine when additional clinical documentation is needed to assign the diagnosis and/or procedure code(s).
3. Consult with physicians and other healthcare providers to obtain further clinical documentation to assist with code assignment.
4. Consult reference materials to facilitate code assignment.
5. Identify patient encounter type.
6. Identify and post charges for healthcare services based on documentation.

Domains II: Diagnosis and Procedure Coding (66%)
Diagnosis

1. Select the diagnoses that require coding according to current coding and reporting requirements for acute care (inpatient) services.
2. Select the diagnoses that require coding according to current coding and reporting requirements for outpatient services.
3. Interpret conventions, formats, instructional notations, tables, and definitions of the classification system to select diagnoses, conditions, problems or other reasons for the encounter that require coding.
4. Sequence diagnoses and other reasons for encounter according to notations and conventions of the classification system and standard data set definitions such as Uniform Hospital Discharge Data Set (UHDDS).
5. Apply the Official ICD-9-CM Coding Guidelines.

Procedure

1. Select the procedures that require coding according to current coding and reporting requirements for acute care (inpatient) services.
2. Select the procedures that require coding according to current coding and reporting requirements for outpatient services.
3. Interpret conventions, formats, instructional notations, and definitions of the classification system or nomenclature to select procedures or services that require coding.
4. Sequence procedures according to notations and conventions of the classification system or nomenclature and standard data set definitions such as UHDDS.
5. Apply the Official ICD-9-CM Coding Guidelines.
6. Apply the official CPT/HCPCS Level II Coding Guidelines.

Domain III: Regulatory Guidelines and Reporting Requirements for Acute-Care (Inpatient) Service (7%)

1. Select the principal diagnosis, principal procedure, complications, comorbid conditions, other diagnoses and procedures that require coding according to UHDDS definitions and *Coding Clinic for ICD-9-CM*.
2. Assign the present on admission (POA) indicators.
3. Evaluate the impact of code selection on diagnosis-related group (DRG) assignment.
4. Verify DRG assignment based on inpatient prospective payment system (IPPS) definitions.
5. Assign or validate the discharge disposition.

Domain IV: Regulatory Guidelines and Reporting Requirements for Outpatient (Ambulatory) Services (7%)

1. Select the reason for encounter, pertinent secondary conditions, primary procedure, and other procedures that require coding according to UHDDS definitions, *CPT Assistant*, and *Coding Clinics for ICD-9-CM*, and HCPCS.
2. Apply outpatient prospective payment system (OPPS) reporting requirements:
   - Modifiers
   - CPT/HCPCS Level II

- Medical necessity
- Evaluation and Management code assignment (facility reporting)
3. Apply clinical laboratory service requirements.

Domain V: Data Quality and Management (3%)

1. Assess the quality of coded data.
2. Communicate with healthcare providers regarding reimbursement methodologies, documentation rules, and regulations related to coding.
3. Analyze health record documentation for quality and completeness of coding.
4. Review the accuracy of abstracted data elements for database integrity and claims processing.
5. Review and resolve coding edits such as Correct Coding Initiative (CCI), Medicare Code Editor (MCE), and Outpatient Code Editor (OCE).

Domain VI: Information and Communication Technologies (2%)

1. Use computer to ensure data collection, storage, analysis, and reporting of information.
2. Use common software applications (for example, word processing, spreadsheets, and e-mail) in the execution of work processes.
3. Use specialized software in the completion of HIM processes.

Domain VII: Privacy, Confidentiality, Legal, and Ethical Issues (3%)

1. Apply policies and procedures for access and disclosure of personal health information.
2. Apply AHIMA Code of Ethics and the Standards of Ethical Coding.
3. Recognize/report privacy issues/problems.
4. Protect data integrity and validity using software or hardware technology.

Domain VIII: Compliance (3%)

1. Evaluate the accuracy and completeness of the patient record as defined by organizational policy and external regulations and standards.
2. Monitor compliance with organization-wide health record documentation and coding guidelines.
3. Recognize and report compliance concerns.

Exam Specifications

The CCS exam consists of the following item types:
- **Theory:** 81 multiple choice theory questions appear first (Domains I, IV–VIII)
- **Application:** 8 multiple select questions (Domain II only)
- **Application:** 12 cases studies (Domain II only)

The total testing time for the CCS exam is 4 hours. Be sure to pace yourself during the exam and use your time wisely.

Instructions and official guidelines for coding medical records are included in the following resources: ICD-9-CM, CPT, UHDDS, *Coding Clinic for ICD-9-CM*, and *CPT Assistant*. However, hospitals and other organizations may develop their own procedures in the absence of approved guidelines. To ensure consistent coding, the specific coding instructions have been developed for use during the CCS exam. The exam coding instructions do not supersede or replace official coding advice and guidelines included in the recommended exam study resources (ahima.org/certification). For Procedures for Coding Medical Record Cases for the CCS Exam, see pages 12–14 in the Introduction of this book.

The Commission on Certification for Health Informatics and Information Management (CCHIIM) manages and sets the strategic direction for the certifications. Pearson Vue is the exclusive provider of AHIMA certification exams. To see sample questions and images of the new exam format, visit ahima.org/certification.

What Books to Bring

For candidates taking the CCS certification exam between **June 1, 2013**, candidates must bring the 2012 or 2013 versions of *ICD-9-CM Volumes 1 through 3*, the 2012 or 2013 HCPCS codebook, and the 2013 American Medical Association *CPT* codebook. (Only the AMA codebook is permitted.) A medical dictionary is optional.

Candidates without the required codebooks will not be permitted to test and will forfeit their application fees. Candidates who do not bring all the required books, or whose books do not have the correct year, will *not* be allowed to test. **For the most up-to-date exam information, visit ahima.org/certification**.

How to Use This Book and Online Assessments

The CCS practice questions and practice exams in this book test knowledge of content pertaining to the CCS competencies published by AHIMA and available at ahima.org/certification. The multiple choice practice questions and practice medical cases along with two practice exams are presented in a similar format to what might be found on the CCS exam.

This book contains a practice section that includes 81 practice multiple choice questions, 8 multiple select questions and seven practice case studies along with two complete practice exams, each comprised of 81 multiple choice questions, 8 multiple select questions and 12 case studies. (Additional coding exercises can also be found in the Introduction of this book.) Each multiple choice question is identified with one of the eight CCS domains, so you will be able to determine whether you need knowledge or skill building in particular areas of the exam domains. The multiple select questions cover only domain II. All answers include rationales and references for further guidance. Pursuing these references will help you build your knowledge and skills in specific domains.

To most effectively use this book, work through all of the practice questions first. This will help you identify areas in which you may need further preparation. For the questions that you answer incorrectly, read the associated references to help refresh your knowledge. After going through the practice questions, take one of the practice exams. Again, for the questions that you answer incorrectly, refresh your knowledge by reading the associated references and study resources.

The online assessments contains the same multiple choice and multiple select questions from the book. The practice questions and practice exams can be presented in random order, or you may choose to go through the questions in sequential order by domain. You may also choose to practice or test your skills on specific domains. For example, if you would like to build your skills in domain II, you may choose only those domains' questions for a given practice session.

About the Online Assessments

The online assessments accompanying this book contains 267 practice multiple choice items covering all eight CCS domains. In addition, there are 31 inpatient and ambulatory case studies.

Introduction

The purpose of this book is to provide practice exercises for the certified coding specialist (CCS) exam through a review of important ICD-9-CM and CPT coding material. Two simulations of the CCS exam are included in this book to help you improve test performance within the context of the four-hour exam. The content of this book is not intended to predict what will be on the CCS exam, and utilizing *CCS Exam Preparation* does not guarantee a passing score. However, *CCS Exam Preparation* does provide a focused method of preparing for the exam through review, practice, and exam simulation.

Steps for Success

1. Review basic coding principals in coding books and then test yourself via the exercises provided in this book and on the accompanying CD.

2. Review relevant American Hospital Association *Coding Clinic* articles. Read as many issues of the *Coding Clinic* as possible but be sure to review the most recent five years (2008 through 2012) beginning with the most recent articles. As noted, the *Coding Clinic* articles used to develop the 2013 CCS exam end with the fourth quarter of 2012. Knowledge of *Coding Clinic* is crucial for success on the CCS exam. Also be sure to review the most recent ICD-9-CM Official Guidelines for Coding and Reporting, which are included in *Coding Clinic*. The national standards for coding practice are provided in *Coding Clinic* and it is therefore the basis for establishing the correct answers related to ICD-9-CM on the CCS exam.

3. Review a CPT educational text and complete exercises for areas in which more skill is needed. Review the guidelines section of each section of the CPT codebook to ensure adequate knowledge of the details of each area.

4. Review the American Medical Association *CPT Assistant* from the most recent issues going backward as far as possible.

5. Complete the introductory exercises and practice questions in this book.

6. To prepare psychologically for the experience of taking the four-hour CCS exam, simulate the experience by completing a practice exam *in one sitting.*

   Along with practice questions and case studies, this book contains two practice exams (each with 81 multiple choice questions, 8 multiple select questions, and 12 cases studies) and additional coding exercises, which appear at the end of this Introduction.

   The online assessment contains three sets of 81 multiple choice practice questions and 8 multiple select questions that can be presented in sequential order (by domain) or random order for a more challenging experience.

7. Follow up with the references and other CCS study resources. *Ask CCS-credentialed professionals for clarification on items that are unclear.*

For more information on the exam, refer to the About the CCS Exam section earlier in this book or visit ahima.org/certification.

Make Plans for CCS Success

In order to develop a good plan of study, it is important to reflect on what you have read so far. Use a calendar to determine how much time you have to prepare.

- How many hours can you spend per week studying?
- How many weeks do you have to study before the exam? (Exclude weeks when you have personal or family events.)

Good preparation using the steps to success can help you achieve a successful exam experience!

Self-Evaluation Notes

Each person who studies for the CCS exam has a different skill set. One of the goals for using this book is to determine your areas of weakness. Strategies can then be developed to make weak areas stronger. Take a few minutes to complete this self-evaluation so that your specific needs can be addressed. Use this self-evaluation to help gather resources before working through the remainder of this book.

I need more practice in these areas:

  1.
  2.
  3.

I can strengthen these areas by:

  1.
  2.
  3.

I need these resources to help me:

  1.
  2.
  3.

Coding Challenges

The following is an outline of potentially challenging coding issues. When possible, obtain the reference materials listed in the back of this book and utilize them. Creating a study schedule and reviewing materials that address your weaknesses will enable you to achieve your goals. Many people find that meeting with a small study group each week in person can help you stay on track. In addition to study group support, there is an AHIMA Community of Practice (CoP), Studying for the CCS, which provides online assistance and resources for members. As you review the different areas of content, identify any weaknesses that you need to focus on for improvement.

In order to do well on the multiple choice section of this book, reference material related to the exam content should be memorized. It is not possible to memorize everything, so developing a study strategy is important. Be sure to read the About the CCS Exam section earlier in this book to fully understand the exam contents and what should be coded in the medical cases. Determine weak areas and study to improve those areas. Focus on clinical scenarios and reimbursement topics that would apply to the "average" hospital.

Codebooks are allowed during the CCS exam. Refer to the AHIMA Certification website (ahima.org/certification) for a current list of allowable codebooks. Furthermore, materials in codebooks must be permanently affixed inside your codebooks. Remember, too, that you will need to gain speed using the codebooks because an encoder is not used to assign codes during the exam. In order to hone this skill, practice coding exercises by timing yourself to evaluate your speed and accuracy using actual codebooks.

The following are highlights to remember:

- Because national coding guidelines and references are used for the CCS exam, evaluate your hospital guidelines to identify any difference between the two. Be sure to code according to national guidelines.

- Recent issues addressed in *Coding Clinic* and CPT Assistant are important. Begin your review from the most recent to the oldest issues. Identify areas that are confusing or have been revised over time. Make sure you understand the most recent decisions regarding any particular coding issue.

- Knowledge of MS-DRGs and APCs are important. Which MS-DRGs will be affected by major comorbidities or complications (MCCs) and complications or comorbidities (CCs) is key information. You should have a general idea about common MS-DRGs for the average hospital in the United States and the reimbursement methodology of APCs. For example, what status indicators mean and how to assign evaluation and management (E/M) levels if given a template.

- An understanding of accurate principal diagnosis assignment is key. It is essential to know the disease processes that underlie ethical coding. Much of this knowledge is based in *Coding Clinic* reference material and the Uniform Hospital Discharge Data Set (UHDDS).

- Generally, cases on the exam reflect common cases that a coder in an average hospital would code. Determine if you have a knowledge deficit in any common coding areas because your facility does not treat that type of patient. For example, some facilities do not provide services for newborns, deliveries, heart catheterizations, coronary artery bypass grafts (CABGs), or neonatal intensive care. If you work in such a facility, you will need to strategize how to gather expertise in these areas. One way to gain expertise is to review the coding exercises in a basic coding book and to use an encoder to determine the MS-DRGs associated with the exercises.

- On the CCS exam, national coding principles are emphasized. Reviewing of the last two years of the *Journal of AHIMA* is a worthwhile endeavor. Be mindful of such topics as future nomenclatures such as ICD-10 and the Health Insurance Portability and Accountability Act (HIPAA). Also, keep in mind that sometimes coders get into habits that may subtly deviate from coding guidelines. Be on alert and identify any of these habits in order to correct them.

ICD-9-CM Review

The following is an outline of some of the more important areas to know.

Infectious Disease

- Review the most recent guidelines regarding sepsis (038.x 1 SIRS code) vs. septicemia (038.x). They require that a code from 038 be used followed by 995.91. If septic shock is also documented, 995.92 and 785.52 should be assigned.

Diabetes

- Review the definition of fifth digits in this category.
- Understand the difference between type I and type II diabetes and the pathophysiology of both types.

Respiratory

- Code for the specific type of pneumonia as documented in the medical record by the provider.
- Know the criteria for recognizing gram-negative and other specific types of pneumonia when documented in the medical record.
- Review the various types of chronic obstructive pulmonary disease (COPD) and how the acute exacerbation of each is coded. Know the criteria for coding asthma with status asthmaticus as specified in *Coding Clinic* and code only when documented in the record.
- Review the criteria for coding respiratory failure and when it may be sequenced first.

Procedures

- Understand how procedures, sometimes performed at the patient's bedside, affect the MS-DRG assignment. Some examples are transbronchial biopsies, ventilator usage, excisional debridement, and tracheostomies.
- Be careful to assign debridement codes appropriately. Do not code an excisional debridement unless there is documentation in the record reflecting that an excisional debridement was performed. Review the *Coding Clinic* guidance associated with excisional debridement.

Gastrointestinal

- Use a combination code whenever available that incorporates a hemorrhage and the specific disorder. Use the 578.x category as an additional code when no combination code has been created or when the cause of the hemorrhage is unknown.
- Understand the difference between a direct (no path report) versus an indirect hernia (path report will show a hernia sac) and how to code them.

Delivery and Pregnancy

- Understand the definition of fifth digits and when to use them. Remember that the fifth digit of 4 is only used for a postpartum complication not in the same episode of the delivery. If you work at a facility that does not perform deliveries, use the review exercises in another coding text to improve your knowledge in this area.
- Memorize the definition of a normal delivery and know the rules for using code 650.
- Recognize that, at a minimum, delivery charts must have the following types of codes: delivery diagnosis code (6xx code), outcome of delivery (V2x.xx), and procedure code (73.59 if no other procedure performed).
- Remember that medical conditions associated with pregnancy, delivery, and puerperium require both a 6xx code as well as a disease code. For example, postpartum anemia is coded as 648.22 and 285.9.

Ectopic Pregnancy and Miscarriages

- Understand the definition of fifth digits and when to use them.
- Understand how to code complications of ectopic pregnancy and abortions during the admission for treatment of the ectopic pregnancy or abortion. Review the Inclusion notes for 639.x category in the ICD Tabular Index and know when to use them.

Anemia

- Review the anemia coding. In particular, there are anemia codes for anemia in chronic illness. Also, blood loss anemia is a commonly associated condition with chronic bleeding and acute bleeding. Be sure to know when to code acute versus chronic blood loss anemia. It is also important to review national guidelines regarding postoperative anemia.

Cardiovascular Conditions

- Remember to specify the location of the myocardial infarction and any comorbidities that will affect the DRG assignment such as arrhythmias, heart failure, hypotension, and so on.
- Review and understand sequencing issues pertaining to arteriosclerotic heart disease (AHD) and unstable angina in *Coding Clinic*.
- Review the coding of cerebral infarctions and sequelae such as aphasia and hemiplegia.
- Review coding cardiac procedures such as cardiac catheterizations and bypass surgery. If you do not have exposure to this type of chart, practice coding these issues using a coding exercise book.

Neoplasms

- Review the definitions of the categories in the table.
  - The primary site is where the cancer arises.
  - A secondary neoplasm is present whenever the neoplasm leaves the organ of origin (where it began). This can occur when the neoplasm travels through the blood and/or the lymphatic system or via direct growth (direct extension) into another adjacent tissue.

- Remember that looking up the morphology type can lead you to the primary site (for example, renal cell carcinoma arises in the kidney).
- Review the suggested steps in *ICD-9-CM Coding Handbook with Answers*, which are synopsized as follows:
  ○ Look up the morphology and code the primary site if given.
  ○ If no primary site code is indicated by the morphology type, the neoplasm table must be used.
  ○ If the term "metastatic" is used ambiguously, assume the following are secondary sites: bone, brain, diaphragm, heart, liver, lymph nodes, mediastinum, meninges, peritoneum, pleura, retroperitoneum, spinal cord, and sites from the 195 category.

Injuries and Burns

- Review the difference between traumatic versus pathological fractures.
- Make sure the most extensive wound is coded and all injured internal organs are coded.
- Review the fifth digits related to intracranial injury, and make sure the appropriate code is used.
- Remember that if burns are located in the same body area, use only the degree of greatest severity. For example, if there are second- and third-degree burns of the forearm, only the third-degree burn of the forearm is coded.

Drugs

- Review the difference between abuse and addiction and the fifth digits associated with them. Also review the coding of procedures associated with this area.
- Review the definition of adverse effect. The following terms indicate an adverse effect of a drug:
  ○ Allergic reaction
  ○ Cumulative effect
  ○ Hypersensitivity
  ○ Idiosyncratic reaction
  ○ Paradoxical reaction
  ○ Synergistic
- Review the definition of poisoning. The following are classified as poisonings when:
  ○ The drug is administered, taken, or prescribed incorrectly, for example, if an overdose of medication occurs
  ○ Alcohol is used in conjunction with a drug
  ○ Street drugs are taken resulting in an overdose or taken in addition to prescribed or over-the-counter (OTC) drugs
  ○ OTC drugs are taken with prescriptions
  ○ Two OTC drugs are used together

Complications

- Review this section of the ICD-9-CM codebook to refresh your memory about how these codes are found.
- Review the Alphabetic and Tabular Indices and what is contained within each category.
- The best way to review this area is to go through the Tabular Index.

- The first area in the Tabular Index contains the three major groupings associated with devices and complications (in the Complications chapter):
  - Mechanical Complications (996.00–996.59)
  - Infection/Inflammation Due to Devices (996.60–996.69)
  - Other Complications (996.70–996.79)
- Review the general complications in the 997 and 998 categories. Remember that a second code is required because of the directions given under the main heading of 997. If the code is not specific to the exact type of complication, a second code should also be used with 998 to denote the specific manifestation. For example, if a patient has intraoperative atrial fibrillation, use 997.1 and 427.31; and if a patient has postoperative septicemia, use 998.59 and 038.9.
- Review the 999 category. Issues such as phlebitis due to IV are listed.
- Complications that occur only in specific body sites are classified in the respective chapter of an ICD-9-CM code book. For example, postoperative pulmonary embolism (415.11) is found in Chapter 7, Diseases of Circulatory System (390–459). Complications of abortion, pregnancy, labor, or delivery are classified to chapter 11, Complications of Pregnancy, Childbirth, and the Puerperium (630–679).

Perinatal Conditions

- Use the V code (V3x.xx) as principal when the admission is for the birth of the infant. Do not use V3x.xx if the admission is not for birth (for example, the patient is transferred).
- Code other perinatal conditions as appropriate such as birth trauma, prematurity, or jaundice when documented in the record.

MS-DRGs and Case Mix

Obtain the MS-DRG list for fiscal year 2013 (refer to the References section in this book). Highlight the most common MS-DRGs that will occur in the average hospital and look at how they are ordered. This type of study will help you become familiar with the most common MS-DRGs and see the hierarchy of MS-DRG decision trees. Generally, the MS-DRG grouper considers the following information: whether the patient had a procedure, the age of the patient, and whether there was a major comorbid condition (MCC).

It is important to review the definitions of case mix and case-mix index (AHIMA 2010, 40–41).

- **Case mix:** 1. A description of a patient population based on any number of specific characteristics, including age, gender, type of insurance, diagnosis, risk factors, treatment received, and resources used

  2. Set of categories of patients (type and volume) treated by a healthcare organization and representing the complexity of the organization's caseload.

- **Case-mix index (CMI):** The average relative weight of all cases treated at a given facility or by a given physician, which reflects the resource intensity or clinical severity of a specific group in relation to the other groups in the classification system; calculated by dividing the sum of the weights of diagnosis-related groups for patients discharged during a given period divided by the total number of patients discharged.

If you do not code inpatient records on a routine basis, it is important to obtain a list of MS-DRGs from the Centers for Medicare and Medicaid Services (CMS 2013, search for *DRG relative weights*). If possible, put some of the exercises or cases in this book into the MS-DRG grouper to familiarize yourself with common MS-DRGs. Switch the principal diagnosis and note how the MS-DRG changes. Also note which MS-DRGs are affected by MCCs.

Review the MS-DRG weights of the most common MS-DRGs that would occur in an average hospital in the United States. The following is a list, which is by no means all-inclusive, of some common clinical scenarios that might form the basis of further study.

Pneumonia
Congestive Heart Failure
Cholecystitis and Cholecystectomy
Malignant Neoplasms with Associated Treatments
    Lung
    Breast
    Prostate
    Colon
Fracture of Femur with Associated Treatments
    Total Hip Replacement
    Open Reduction with Internal Fixation
Septicemia
Gastrointestinal Hemorrhage
COPD with Exacerbation
Respiratory Failure
Deliveries
Newborns
Anemia

Review the common MS-DRGs that cannot be optimized unless a procedure is found or the principal diagnosis is changed. Try to find some examples.

Use a grouper that you have access to in your work or academic institution or use a free DRG grouper (for example, from irp.com). *Disclaimer: This software application may contain errors and is not endorsed or developed by the author or AHIMA.*

Case-mix Exercises

The following exercises are meant to help you learn more about case-mix analysis and increase your knowledge of MS-DRGs. In actual coding practice, it would only be appropriate to switch the principal diagnoses if the clinical information conformed to UHDDS guidelines that supported a change in principal diagnosis. Try the following exercises. The discharge disposition is discharged to home.

1. A 22-month-old child has pyelonephritis (590.80) and dehydration (276.51) and both are equally treated. Which MS-DRG will have the highest weight?

2. If a 65-year-old patient has pneumonia (486) and congestive heart failure (428.0), which DRG will have a higher weight?

3. If a 70-year-old patient has pneumonia due to *Escherichia coli* (482.82) and an acute exacerbation of COPD (491.21), which DRG will have a higher weight?

4. Case mix (CM) and case-mix index (CMI) calculations: The CM is all of the weights added together. The CMI is the average weight of all the cases in a given dataset or period of time. What is the case mix and CMI for these cases using the highest paying MS-DRGs?

Answers are in the Answer Key in the back of this book.

CPT Review

Review the beginning of each section in the CPT code book for instructions about definitions and other information pertinent to assigning the correct code. The following are points to review:

Integumentary (Skin)

- Review the section on lacerations (repair) in the CPT book regarding when to add the lengths together and when to use an addition code for closure of the wound.
- Remember that grafts are measured in square centimeters, which is different than lacerations.
- Review the use of codes involved in excision, destruction, or other methods of removing lesions in the Malignant, Benign, Skin Tags, Other Lesions section.

Endoscopies

- In general, the Alphabetical Index will provide a range of codes for a given procedure. Some of these are open procedures. Make sure you look up each code before assigning it.
- There is a difference between "brushings and washings" and a biopsy in CPT.
  - Review the definitions of upper and lower gastrointestinal (GI) endoscopies in CPT
  - Upper gastrointestinal endoscopy
  - Proctosigmoidoscopy
  - Sigmoidoscopy
  - Colonoscopy
  - Review the Laparoscopy section of CPT
  - Review the definitions of the sinus procedures
  - Review the definitions under bronchoscopies. Remember that a bilateral bronchoscopy is coded twice or with a –50 modifier.

Musculoskeletal

- Review the terminology differences between ICD and CPT related to the treatment of fractures. For example, "manipulation" is the same in CPT as "reduction" in ICD-9.
- Understand the medical terminology, approaches, notes, and inclusions for knee repairs.

Outpatient Prospective Payment System

The outpatient prospective payment system (OPPS), for ambulatory care, began to be used for Medicare in August 2000. This system uses the ambulatory payment classifications (APCs) for reimbursement for hospital-based outpatient services such as outpatient surgery, emergency department visits, outpatient clinic visits, and outpatient ancillary tests. Some highlights of this system are listed here:

- APCs are similar to MS-DRGs in that they are both prospective payment methodologies and both have relative weights.
- APCs are different from MS-DRGs because outpatients can have multiple APCs for a given encounter, whereas an inpatient can have only one MS-DRG.
- APCs are generated for many services, such as x-rays, medical tests, clinic or emergency visits, surgical procedures, devices, drugs and biologicals, and partial hospitalizations.
- The billing number is the connecting identifier for a given patient's encounter that results in multiple APCs.

Status indicators denote what type of service was provided and assist in determining the payment. Status indicators include: X, ancillary; V, clinic or emergency department visit; T, significant procedure that is discounted when other T procedures are provided (the first procedure is paid at a rate of 100 percent whereas the second and those thereafter are paid at 50 percent); S, significant procedure that is paid at 100 percent and is not discounted; P, partial hospitalization; H, Pass-through device categories; G/J, drugs/biologicals; K, Non-pass-through drugs and nonimplantable biological, including therapeutic radiopharmaceuticals. Please visit the CMS web page (noted in the References in this book) for more information and a complete list of status indicators.

- CPT (numeric) and HCPCS (alphanumeric) modifiers approved for hospital outpatient are listed on the CPT codebook inside cover; –25,–27,–50, –52, –58, –59, –73, –74, –76, –77, –78, –79, –91, –LT, –RT, –CA, –CR, –E1, –E2, –E3, –E4, –FA, –FB, –FC –F1, –F2, –F3, –F4, –F5, –F6, –F7, –F8, –F9, –GA, –GG, –GH, –LC, –LD,–Q0, –Q1, –QM, –QN, –RC, –TA, –T1, –T2, –T3, –T4, –T5, –T6, –T7, –T8, –T9.

- The following is a *hypothetical* example of one patient's APCs for a given encounter in the emergency department.

Billing Number	Status Indicator	CPT/HCPC	APC	Amount
789321	V	99284–25	0615	$223.17
789321	T	25500	0129	$111.73
789321	X	72050	0261	$75.23
789321	S	72128	0332	$195.07
789321	S	70450	0332	$195.07
			Reimbursement Total =	$800.27

While reviewing *Coding Clinic* and *CPT Assistant*, keep three goals in mind:

- Review the past three to five years of both references to prepare for the multiple choice and coding sections of the examination. Review at least the past three years of both references beginning with the most recent issue and reading backward (for instance, read 4th Quarter 2012, then 3rd Quarter 2012). This will allow you to know when changes occurred and what the most recent requirements are.

- Review as many topics that pertain to common inpatient and outpatient diagnoses and procedures for services that the average hospital would provide as you can. Be sure to read the fiscal year (FY) 2012 Official Coding Guidelines.

- Bolster knowledge in your areas of weakness that you have identified. The references used to develop the 2013 CCS exam stop at the end of 2012.

Ambulatory Payment Classifications (APCs)

It is important to understand the methodology of APCs. Some important issues to review are discounting, impact of CPT and HCPCS codes, medical necessity, the Correct Coding Initiative (CCI), status indicators, packaging, and the three-year transitional corridor. Refer to the Coding Challenges later in this section. AHIMA also has excellent resources regarding this topic. Also visit the CMS website for Medicare Program Memorandum.

Health Insurance Portability and Accountability Act (HIPAA)

Review recent AHIMA Practice Briefs and articles on this topic. Questions about HIPAA could be present on the exam. An easy way to study this area is to access information from the Body of Knowledge from the AHIMA CoP.

Common Diseases and Disorders with Associated Drugs

This is *not* a comprehensive list but can be helpful for review.

AIDS—Immunodeficiency syndrome caused by the human immunodeficiency virus (HIV). This disorder is associated with opportunistic infections, malignancies, and neurologic disease.
Medications: NRTIs-Nucleoside Reverse Transcriptase Inhibitors (Retrovir, AZT, Videx, ddl, Hivid, ddC, Zeril, d4tT, Epivir, 3TC, Emtricitabine, Tenofovir, Zidovudine); NRTIs-Nonnucleoside Reverse Transcriptase Inhibitors (Viramunde, Sustiva, Delavirdine, Rilpivirine, Etravirine, Nevirapine); Protease Inhibitors; (Invirase, Saquinavir, Crixovan, Indinavir, Kaletra, Lipinavir, Ritinavir, Atazanavir, Darunavir, Prezista, Tibotec, Fosamprenavir, Lexiva)

Allergies—Hypersensitivity to a substance that does not normally cause a reaction.
Medications: antihistamines such as Claritin, Phenergan, Allegra, Zyrtec. The most common antihistamine for allergic reaction is diphenhydramine (Benadryl)

Anemia—Reduction in the number of circulating red blood cells or a reduction in the amount of hemoglobin in each red blood cell.
Medications: iron supplements, ferrous sulfate (Feosol), ferrous fumarate (Femiron), ferrous gluconate (Fergon); B_{12} (Cyanocobalamin); hematopoietic agents (Procrit, Epogen, Neupogen)

Angina pectoris—Severe pain associated with constriction in blood vessels to the heart with pain radiating to the left arm, abdomen, back, or jaw.
Medications: verapamil (Verelan, Calan SR); diltiazem (Cardizem CD, Dilacor); nifedipine (Adalat, Procardia); nitrates (Isordil, Imdur, ISMO); NTG-nitroglycerin (Nitroquick, Nitro-Dur); atenolol (Tenormin)

Anxiety—Mental disorder that manifests as fear, worry, or dread that is not related to a specific event or set of objects.
Medications: lorazepam (Ativan); alprazolam (Xanax); diazepam (Valium); paroxetine (Paxil); buspirone (Buspar); citalopram HBr (Celexa), fluoxetine Hcl (Prozac), sertraline (Zoloft), escitalopram (Lexapro)

Arrhythmia—Irregularities in the force or rhythm of the heart such as atrial fibrillation, tachycardia, bradycardia, or cardiac arrest.
Medications: verapamil (Calan SR, Verelan); digoxin (Lanoxin); quinidine (Quinaglute, Quinidex); amiodarone (Cordarone)

Arthritis—Inflammation of the joints. There are three major types of arthritis: osteoarthritis, rheumatoid arthritis, and gout.
Medications: ibuprofen (Advil, Motrin); hydrocortisone; Lodine; naproxen (Naprosyn); Oruvail; prednisone (Deltasone); Relafen; Voltaren; Medrol; Daypro; Celebrex

Asthma—Spasm of the bronchial tubes or swelling of the mucous membrane.
Medications: albuterol (Proventil, Ventolin); theophylline; Theo-Dur; Serevent; Xopenex; Azmacort; Atrovent

Bipolar disorder—Mental disorder in which both mania and depression occur.
Medications: lithium; Lithobid; Eskalith; Zyprexa

Chronic obstructive pulmonary disease (COPD)—Group of disorders that decrease the ability of the lungs to provide ventilation to the body. Some forms of COPD include chronic obstructive asthma, chronic obstructive bronchitis, emphysema, bronchiectasis, and combinations of the aforementioned disorders.
Medications: Prednisone, albuterol (Proventil, Ventolin); Serevent; Alupent; Atrovent

Congestive heart failure (CHF)—Inability of the heart to pump the blood through the body adequately, resulting in edema in the extremities.
Medications: Amiloride (Midamor), Bumetanide (Bumex), Chlorothiazide (Diuril), Chlorthalidone (Hygroton), Furosemide (Lasix), Hydro-chlorothiazide (Esidrix, Hydrodiuril), Indapamide (Lozol), Spironolactone (Aldactone), Benazepril Lotensin), Captopril (Capoten), Enalapril (Vasotec), Fosinopril (Monopril, Lisinopril (Prinivil, Zestril), Moexipril (Univasc), Perindopril (Aceon), Quinapril (Accupril), Ramipril (Altace), Trandolapril (Mavik), Acebutolol (Sectral), Atenolol (Tenormin), Betaxolol (Kerlone), Bisoprolol/hydrochlorothiazide (Ziac), Bisoprolol (Zebeta), Carteolol (Cartrol), Metoprolol (Lopressor, Toprol XL), Nadolol (Corgard), Propranolol (Inderal), Sotalol (Betapace), Timolol (Blocadren)

Dehydration—Loss of body fluid; this may be associated with severe nausea and vomiting, diarrhea, high fever, and urinary tract infections.
Medications: intravenous fluids, oral fluids; Pedialyte; Infalyte; Gatorade; Sportade

Depression—Mental disorder in which there is loss of interest in usually pleasurable pursuits.
Medications: amitriptyline hydrochloride (Elavil); Celexa; nortriptyline hydrochloride (Pamelor); Paxil; Prozac; trazodone hydrochloride (Desyrel); Zoloft

Diabetes mellitus—Disorder in which there is inadequate production or utilization of insulin. There are two types: Type I (the body does not produce or does not produce enough endogenous insulin) and type II (the cells of the body do not utilize the endogenous insulin properly).
Medications: glyburide (DiaBeta, Glynase PresTab, Micronase); Glucophage; Glucotrol; insulin (Humulin, Humalog, Novolin), Lantus, Metformin, Glucophage XR, Fortamet, Glumetza

Diverticulitis—Infection of the diverticula that causes inflammation.
Medications: antibiotics: ampicillin; gentamicin; tetracycline; cephalosporins (Mefoxin, Rocephin, Fortaz)

Diverticulosis—Formation of diverticula in the large intestine that can bleed or become infected or inflamed.
Medications: High-fiber diet

Fever—Elevated temperature.
Medications: acetaminophen (Tylenol); aspirin; ibuprofen (Motrin, Advil, Nuprin)

Gastrointestinal ulcers—Lesion in the mucosal membrane of the gastrointestinal tract that may cause bleeding or perforation. When a perforation occurs, the bacteria in the gastrointestinal tract may spill into the adjacent body cavity, causing peritonitis.
Medications: Axid; Nexium; Pepcid; Prilosec; Tagamet; Zantac

Hyperlipidemia—Excessive amount of lipids (fat) in the blood.
Medications: gemfibrozil (Lopid, Mevacor, Pravachol, Zocor, Lipitor)

Hypertension—Blood pressure that is persistently higher than normal. Malignant hypertension is characterized by severe vascular and other internal organ damage.
Medications: Altace; atenolol (Tenormin); Accupril; Capoten; Cardura; Coreg; Corgard; DynaCirc; enalapril (Vasotec); Hytrin; Lotensin; metropolol (Lopressor); Norvasc; Prinivil; Zestril, Benazepril (Lotensin), Fosinopril (Monopril), Lisinopril, Moexipril (Univasc),Perindopril (Aceon),Quinapril (Accupril),Ramipril (Altace),Trandolapril (Mavik), Acebutolol (Sectral), Atenolol (Tenormin),Betaxolol (Kerlone), Bisoprolol/hydrochlorothiazide (Ziac),Bisoprolol (Zebeta),Carteolol (Cartrol), Toprol XL,Nadolol,Propranolol (Inderal),Sotalol (Betapace),Timolol (Blocadren)

Hypokalemia—Potassium depletion in the blood.
Medications: potassium chloride (K-Dur, K-Lyte, Micro-K, Klor-Con, K-Tab, Kaon, K-Lor)

Hypotension—Persistently lower-than-normal blood pressure. There are two common forms of hypotension: orthostatic and that due to other disorders such as anemia, trauma, hemorrhage, and fever.
Medications: volume expansion by increasing salt (NaCl); fludrocortisone acetate (Florinef Acetate); ephedrine

Hypothyroid—Decreased amount of thyroid secretion.
Medications: Levoxyl; Synthroid; thyroid; Levothroid; Cytomel

Impotence—Inability to maintain or achieve erection. This can occur because of an organic cause: following a radical prostatectomy, due to diabetes or alcohol abuse, or due to medications. Psychological reasons can also be a cause of this disorder.
Medications: Viagra; Cialis, Levitra, alprostadil (Muse, Edex, Caverject)

Infections—Result of an invasion of a pathogenic agent such as a virus or a bacterium. Infectious organisms include: bacteria (such as streptococci, staphylococci, spirochetes), viruses, fungi, and protozoa.
Medications: antibiotics; amoxicillin trihydrate (Amoxil); ampicillin; Augmentin; Bactroban; Beepen-VK; Biaxin; Ceclor; Ceftin; Cefzil; cephalexin; Cipro; Claforan; Cotrim; doxycycline; Duricef; erythromycin (E.E.S., E-Mycin 333, Erythrocin, EryTab); Floxin; Fortaz; Lorabid; Macrobid; neomycin and polymixin; Penicillin VK; Pen-Vee K; Peridex; Principen; Rocephin; Suprax; tetracycline; Trimox; Vantin; Veetids; Zithromax; antifungals; Diflucan; Lotrisone; Nizoral; nystatin; antivirals; famvir; Valtrex; metronidazole; Zovirax

Malignant neoplasms—Uncontrolled growth of cells and the dispersion of malignant cells through the blood, the lymph system, or by direct extension to tissue adjacent to the tumor.
Medications: chemotherapy; 5-Fluorouracil; chlorambucil; cisplatin (Platinol); Cytoxan; doxorubicin (Adriamycin); Flutamide, megestrol acetate (Megace), MTX-methotrexate; prednisone; Taxol; Taxotere; vinblastine (Velban); vincristine (Oncovin); hormonal therapy; Arimidex; goserelin (Zoladex); Lupron; Proscar; Tamoxifen; biological response modifiers; Herceptin; Intron; Proleukin, IL-2; Roferon

Pneumonia or pneumonitis—Infection or inflammation of the lungs. There are multiple causes such as infectious agents (bacterial or virus), aspiration of secretions or food, inhalation of fumes, or radiation.
Medications: See Infections

Septicemia—Systemic infection usually manifesting in pathogenic organisms or accumulation of their toxins in the bloodstream.
Medications: See Infections

Thrombophlebitis—Inflammation of a vein. This condition leaves the patient at risk for embolisms.
Medication: warfarin sodium (Coumadin); heparin

Schizophrenia—Group of disorders characterized by disordered thinking, effect, and behavior.
Medications: haloperidol (Haldol); chlorpromazine (Thorazine); thioridazine (Mellaril); fluphenazine (Prolixin); Serentil; Seroquel; Clozaril; Zyprexa

Seizure—Involuntary muscular contractions and relaxations.
Medications: Depakote; Dilantin; Klonopin; Neurontin; phenobarbital; Tegretol; diazepam (Valium); Topamax

Procedures for Coding Medical Record Cases for the CCS Examination

Instructions and official guidelines for coding medical records are included in the following resources: *ICD-9-CM*, *CPT*, UHDDS, *Coding Clinic for ICD-9-CM* and *CPT Assistant*. However, hospitals and other organizations may develop their own procedures in the absence of approved guidelines. To ensure consistent coding, the following procedures have been developed for use in the CCS examination. The procedures do not supersede or replace official coding advice and guidelines included in the resources identified above.

These procedures are to be used only in completing the CCS examination. They will be provided to test takers as part of the examination packet. Not adhering to these procedures may result in the miscoding of an exercise, which may result in the deduction of points when the item is scored.

Inpatient Coding

1. Apply UHDDS definitions, ICD-9-CM instructional notations and conventions, and current approved national ICD-9-CM coding guidelines to assign correct ICD-9-CM diagnostic and procedural codes to hospital inpatient medical records.

2. Sequence the ICD-9-CM codes, listing the principal diagnosis first.

3. Code other diagnoses that coexist at the time of admission, that develop subsequently, or that affect the treatment received and/or the length of stay. These represent additional conditions that affect patient care in terms of requiring clinical evaluation, therapeutic treatment, diagnostic procedures, extended length of hospital stay, or increased nursing care and/or monitoring.

   a. Code diagnoses that require active intervention during hospitalization. For example: Admission for small-bowel ileus and subsequent aspiration pneumonia that is treated with antibiotics and respiratory therapy. Code the ileus and aspiration pneumonia.

   b. Code diagnoses that require active management of chronic disease during hospitalization, which is defined as a patient who is continued on chronic management at time of hospitalization. For example: Admission for acute exacerbation of COPD. The patient has depression that extends the stay and for which psychiatric consultation is obtained. Code the COPD and depression. For example: Admission for acute exacerbation of COPD. Physician lists "history of depression" on face sheet, and the patient is given Desyrel. Code the COPD and depression.

   c. Code diagnoses of chronic systemic or generalized conditions that are not under active management when a physician documents them in the record and that may have a bearing on the management of the patient. For example: Admission for breast mass; diagnosis is carcinoma. Patient is blind and requires increased care. Code the breast carcinoma and blindness.

   d. Code status post previous surgeries or conditions likely to recur that may have a bearing on the management of the patient. For example: Admission for pneumonia; status post-cardiac bypass surgery. Code the pneumonia and status post-cardiac bypass surgery (V code).

   e. Do not code status post previous surgeries or histories of conditions that have no bearing on the management of the patient. For example: Admission for pneumonia; status post-hernia repair six months prior to admission. Code only the pneumonia. Previous surgeries involving transplants, internal devices, and prosthetics should be coded.

   f. Do not code localized conditions that have no bearing on the management of the patient. For example: Admission for hernia repair; the patient has a nevus on his leg that is not treated or evaluated. Code only the hernia and its repair.

g. Do not code abnormal findings (laboratory, x-ray, pathologic, and other diagnostic results) unless there is documentary evidence from the physician of their clinical significance. For example: Admission for elective joint replacement for degenerative joint disease. The laboratory report shows a serum sodium of 133; no further documentation addresses this laboratory result. Code only the degenerative joint disease and the replacement surgery. For example: Admission for elective joint replacement for degenerative joint disease. The laboratory report shows a low potassium level, and the physician documents hypokalemia. Intravenous potassium was administered by the physician for hypokalemia. Code the degenerative joint disease, the replacement surgery, and hypokalemia.

h. Do not code symptoms and signs that are characteristic of a diagnosis. For example: A patient has dyspnea due to COPD. Code only the COPD.

i. Do not code condition(s) in the Social History section that has no bearing on the management of the patient.

4. Do not assign E codes, except those that identify the causative substance for an adverse effect of a drug that is correctly prescribed and properly administered and/or poisoning (E850–E949).

5. Do not assign Morphology codes (M codes).

6. Code all procedures that fall within the code range 00.01–86.99, but do not code 57.94 (Foley catheter).

7. Do not code procedures that fall within the code range 87.01–99.99. But code procedures in the following ranges:

87.51–87.54, Cholangiograms

87.74 and 87.76, Retrogrades, urinary systems

88.40–88.58, Arteriography and angiography

92.21–92.29, Radiation therapy

94.24–94.27, Psychiatric therapy

94.61–94.69, Alcohol/drug detoxification and rehabilitation.

96.04, Insertion of endotracheal tube

96.56, Other lavage of bronchus and trachea

96.70–96.72, Mechanical ventilation

98.51–98.59, ESWL

99.25, Chemotherapy

Ambulatory Care Coding

1. Apply ICD-9-CM instructional notations and conventions and current approved Diagnostic Coding and Reporting Guidelines for Outpatient Services (Section IV of the official ICD-9-CM Guidelines for Coding and Reporting),to select diagnoses, conditions, problems, or other reasons for care that require ICD-9-CM coding in an ambulatory care encounter/visit either in a hospital clinic, outpatient surgical area, emergency room, physician's office, or other ambulatory care setting.

2. Sequence the ICD-9-CM code so that the first diagnosis shown in the medical record is the one chiefly responsible for the outpatient services provided during the encounter/visit.

3. Code the secondary diagnoses as follows:

a. Chronic diseases that are treated on an ongoing basis may be coded and reported as many times as the patient receives treatment and care for the condition(s).

b. Code all documented conditions that coexist at the time of the encounter/visit that require or affect patient care, treatment, or management.

c. Conditions previously treated and no longer existing should not be coded.

4. Do not assign E codes, except those that identify the causative substance for an adverse effect of a drug that is correctly prescribed and properly administered and/or poisoning (E850–E949).

5. Do not assign Morphology codes (M codes).

6. Do not assign ICD-9-CM procedure codes.

7. Assign CPT codes for all surgical procedures that fall in the surgery section.

8. Assign CPT codes from the following ONLY IF indicated on the case cover sheet:

    a. Anesthesia section

    b. Medicine section

    c. Evaluation and management services section

    d. Radiology section

    e. Laboratory and pathology section

9. Assign CPT/HCPCS modifiers for hospital-based facilities, if applicable (regardless of payer).

10. Do not assign HCPCS Level II (alphanumeric) codes.

Evaluation and Management Mapping

The following map shows how a given facility has determined the criteria for evaluation and management (E/M) code assignment based on an emergency department record. Use the map to determine the correct codes for the emergency record that is provided. *Remember that each facility has the ability to develop its own mapping strategy. Therefore, the mapping scenario for the CCS exam will most likely be different from this one.* The purpose of this exercise is to practice using any mapping criteria that you are provided during the national exam. The following are the points need to determine the level of CPT code:

Level 1 = 1–20

Level 2 = 21–35

Level 3 = 36–47

Level 4 = 48–60

Level 5 = > 61

Critical Care > 61 with constant physician attendance

CPT Codes

Level 1 99281 99281–25 with procedure/laboratory/radiology

Level 2 99282 99282–25 with procedure/laboratory/radiology

Level 3 99283 99283–25 with procedure/laboratory/radiology

Level 4 99284 99284–25 with procedure/laboratory/radiology

Level 5 99285 99285–25 with procedure/laboratory/radiology

Emergency Department Acuity Points					
	5	10	15	20	25
Meds Given	0–2	3–5	6–7	8–9	> 10
Extent of Hx	Brief	PF	EPF	Detail	Comprehensive
Extent of Exam	Brief	PF	EPF	Detail	Comprehensive
Number of Tests Ordered	0–1	2–3	4–5	6–7	> 8
Supplies Used	1	2–3	4–5	6–7	> 8

E/M MAPPING EXERCISE—EMERGENCY DEPARTMENT RECORD

DATE OF ADMISSION: 6/19   **DATE OF DISCHARGE:**   6/19

HISTORY (Problem Focused):

ADMISSION HISTORY: This 45-year-old African-American male was working in his office when he received news that his daughter, who is in the military, was deployed emergently to the Middle East. He began to have sharp pain in his right chest.

ALLERGIES: None

CHRONIC MEDICATIONS: None

FAMILY HISTORY: Noncontributory

SOCIAL HISTORY: The patient smokes one pack of cigarettes per day, but he does not smoke in the house.

REVIEW OF SYSTEMS: His integumentary, musculoskeletal, cardiovascular, genitourinary, and gastrointestinal systems are negative.

PHYSICAL EXAMINATION (Extended Problem Focused):

   GENERAL APPEARANCE: This is an alert cooperative male in acute distress.

   HEENT: PERRLA, extraocular movements are full

   NECK: Supple

   CHEST: Lungs are clear without rales or rhonchi. Heart has normal sinus rhythm.

   ABDOMEN: Soft and nontender, no organomegaly

   EXTREMITIES: Examination is normal

   LABORATORY DATA: Urinalysis is normal, EKG normal, chest x-ray is normal. CBC and diff, cardiac enzymes show no abnormalities.

IMPRESSION: Noncardiac chest pain

TREATMENT: Patient was reassured, counseled to stop smoking, and referred to the clinic for smoking cessation and further management.

DISCHARGE DIAGNOSES: Noncardiac chest pain, possible anxiety reaction, smoking

DISCHARGE INSTRUCTIONS: The patient was instructed to make an appointment for the clinic tomorrow.

Answer the following questions:

   1. What is the diagnostic code?
   2. Based on the mapping scenario, what CPT code should be used?

(Answers can be found in the Answer Key in the back of this book.)

Coding Exercises

Code these cases in accordance with the exam coding instruction requirements listed earlier.

Inpatient

1. Admission for inguinal hernia repair. This 30-year-old patient has acquired immunodeficiency syndrome (AIDS) but is not symptomatic due to medication regimen. The procedure performed was a right indirect inguinal herniorrhaphy.

2. A 75-year-old male patient was admitted from a nursing home with dehydration and dysphagia due to a previous stroke. During hospitalization the patient was rehydrated and transferred back to the nursing home.

3. A patient is admitted to an acute care facility for detoxification from alcohol intoxication and barbiturate abuse with chronic alcoholism and barbiturate abuse. The patient also has cirrhosis of the liver due to alcoholism.

4. A 30-year-old patient was seen in the emergency department for repetitive epileptic seizures. The patient also had tic douloureux.

5. A patient was admitted to an acute care facility with a temperature of 102 and atrial fibrillation. The chest x-ray reveals pneumonia with subsequent documentation by the physician of pneumonia in the progress notes and discharge summary. The patient was treated with oral antiarrhythmia medications and IV antibiotics.

6. A patient with chronic cholecystitis and gallbladder stones underwent a laparoscopic cholecystectomy in an acute care facility. However, due to extensive gallbladder adhesions the procedure was converted to an open cholecystectomy.

7. A patient is admitted to the inpatient setting with hydronephrosis and a staghorn calculus of the kidney. The patient underwent an ureteroscopy with placement of ureteral stents and removal of calculus.

8. A 77-year-old nursing home patient was admitted to the acute care setting for excisional debridement of decubitus ulcer of the heel via surgical excision in the OR. The patient also has degenerative joint disease of both knees.

9. A 45-year-old woman was admitted to the inpatient setting for a displacement of a lumbar intervertebral disk. This was treated with a laminectomy and diskectomy.

10a. A 34-year-old woman delivered a live born, term baby boy with macrosomia. She had a hemorrhage following an episiotomy with a low forceps delivery but prior to expulsion of the placenta.

10b. A single, newborn, term live-born baby boy.

11. Twin newborns, both born prematurely at 32 weeks via cesarean section, 1,002 g was the birth weight of the first twin, whose mate was stillborn. The baby was admitted to the nursery from the delivery room. The baby also was treated for jaundice due to ABO incompatibility.

12. A patient is admitted to the acute care facility with chest pain. The patient was awakened from sleep; this was the patient's first experience with chest pain. The patient was given two nitroglycerin tablets in the emergency department. The chest pain was not relieved, resulting in the diagnosis of new onset unstable angina. Serial CPK was normal. Following a left cardiac catheterization and coronary angiography, the patient is found to have arteriosclerotic coronary artery disease.

13. This is the first admission for a patient with adenocarcinoma of the right lower lung who was also found with metastasis to the brain. The patient underwent a right lower lung lobectomy.

14. A patient has metastatic adenocarcinoma of bone.

15. A patient is admitted with metastatic carcinoma from breast to liver with previous mastectomy and no reoccurrence at the primary site.

16. A young woman was admitted after a car hit her from behind while she waited for a bus. She sustained a fractured fibula shaft and patella with a break in the skin at the midcalf. The patient required an open reduction of the fibula fracture.

17. Syncope; bradycardia ruled out; due to taking Valium as prescribed by a physician. Patient also took an antihistamine as directed on the package without consulting a healthcare provider.

18. Sepsis due to the presence of an indwelling urinary catheter with a positive blood culture reflected in the progress notes of *Staphylococcus aureus* sepsis.

19. Respiratory distress syndrome, 26-day-old baby, temporary tracheotomy completed.

Ambulatory/Outpatient

20. Noncardiac chest pain, esophageal acid reflux test.
21. Annual screening mammogram.
22. Excision of basal cell carcinoma, 1.9-cm lesion left upper eyelid.
23. Hallux valgus repair with resection of the joint with implant in the first left toe proximal phalanx.
24. Metastatic ovarian cancer to the pleura. Thoracoscopic pleurodesis.
25. Symptomatic bradycardia due to sick sinus syndrome with replacement of dual chamber pacemaker generator with removal of old generator.
26. Esophagogastroduodenoscopy with sclerotherapy of esophageal varices.
27. Transurethral resection of the prostate for benign prostatic hypertrophy with electrocautery.
28. Cryosurgical destruction of simple papilloma of the penis.
29. Dysfunctional uterine bleeding for which hysteroscopy with endometrial ablation was undertaken.
30. Incompetent cervix with removal of cervical cerclage under spinal anesthesia in a pregnant woman.

PRACTICE QUESTIONS

A blank answer sheet for these multiple choice questions can be found on page 46.

Domain I *Health Information Documentation*

1. An 84-year-old woman was admitted and discharged with hemiplegia and aphasia. A CT scan of the brain was performed that revealed an acute cerebral infarction and a possible small brain mass. After further testing, the patient was discharged with a final diagnosis of acute cerebral infarction. The condition(s) that should be coded are:

   a. Acute cerebral infarction

   b. Hemiplegia and aphasia

   c. Acute cerebral infarction, hemiplegia, and aphasia

   d. Possible brain mass, hemiplegia, and aphasia

2. A patient is discharged with a diagnosis of acute pulmonary edema due to congestive heart failure. What condition(s) should be coded?

   a. Acute pulmonary edema

   b. Congestive heart failure

   c. Acute pulmonary edema and congestive heart failure

   d. Unable to determine based on the information provided

3. The patient was admitted from the emergency department because of chest pain. Following blood work, it was determined that the patient had elevated CPKs and MB enzymes. The EKG shows nonspecific ST changes. What type of diagnosis might this indicate?

   a. Unstable angina

   b. Myocardial infarction

   c. Congestive heart failure

   d. Mitral valve stenosis

4. A patient is admitted and diagnosed with a fever and urinary burning. The discharge diagnosis is *Eschericia coli*, urosepsis. Which of the following represents the correct diagnoses and appropriate sequence of those conditions?

   a. Fever, urinary burning, urosepsis

   b. Fever, urinary burning, sepsis

   c. *Eschericia coli*, urinary tract infection

   d. Urinary tract infection, *Eschericia coli*

5. A patient was admitted with heart failure within one week of a heart transplant. Due to the timing, the coder thought that it may represent a postoperative transplant rejection following heart transplant. What action(s) should the coding staff take?

   a. Query the physician.

   b. Assign the codes for the postoperative transplant rejection.

   c. Assign only the code for the transplant rejection.

   d. Assign only the code for heart failure.

6. A patient is admitted to a psychiatric unit of an acute-care facility. The patient experienced the following symptoms almost every day for the last month: loss of interest or pleasure in most or all activities, which is a change from her prior level of functioning. She has also gained 15 lbs, has difficulty falling asleep, feels fatigued, and has difficulty making decisions. What potential diagnosis most closely fits the patient's overall symptoms?

    a. Insomnia

    b. Major depression

    c. Reye's syndrome

    d. Bipolar disorder

7. A patient is admitted to the hospital complaining of abdominal pain. Following evaluation, it was determined that the patient had an intestinal obstruction due to adhesions from a prior abdominal surgery. The patient underwent an exploratory laparotomy with lysis of adhesions. What conditions should be coded?

    a. Abdominal pain, abdominal adhesions, abdominal obstruction, laparotomy, lysis of adhesions

    b. Abdominal adhesions, abdominal obstruction, postoperative complications of the digestive system, laparotomy, lysis of adhesions

    c. Abdominal adhesions with obstruction, lysis of adhesions

    d. Abdominal adhesions and abdominal obstruction, postoperative complications of the digestive system, lysis of adhesions

8. A patient has a principal diagnosis of pneumonia (486) (MS-DRG 195). Which of the following may legitimately change the coding of the pneumonia in accordance with the UHDDS and relevant clinical documentation?

    a. Sputum culture reflects growth of normal flora.

    b. Patient has a positive gram stain.

    c. Patient is found to have dysphagia with aspiration.

    d. Patient has nonproductive sputum.

9. A patient is diagnosed with infertility due to endometriosis and undergoes a laparoscopic laser destruction of pelvic endometriosis. In order to code this encounter accurately, what steps must the coder take?

    a. Review the operative report to determine what procedure codes to use and also to determine the site or sites of endometriosis so codes with the highest specificity may be assigned, and use infertility as a principal diagnosis.

    b. Review the operative report to determine where the laser was used in the pelvis so the site or sites of endometriosis can be specified, and assign a principal diagnosis of infertility.

    c. Review the operative report to determine where the laser was used in the pelvis so the site or sites of endometriosis can be specified as principal, and assign a secondary diagnosis of infertility.

    d. Review the operative report to determine what procedure codes to use and also to determine the site or sites of endometriosis so codes with the highest specificity may be assigned, and use the diagnosis of infertility as a secondary condition.

10. In order to establish the adequacy of documentation the following must be reflected:

    a. Decisions of patient's caregivers

    b. Quantitative analysis of the number of pages

    c. Ancillary forms and consents

    d. Care rendered to the patient and the patient's response

11. Authentication of health record entries means to:

    a. Create facsimiles of documents

    b. Prove authorship of documents

    c. Develop documents

    d. Use a rubber stamp on random sets of documents

12. The requirements for documentation and record completion (documents such as history and physicals, discharge summaries, and consultations) as well as penalties for nonadherence must be specified in:

    a. Hospital rules and regulations

    b. Conditions of nonparticipation

    c. Medical staff bylaws

    d. Nursing staff policies

Domain II *Diagnosis & Procedure Coding*

13. A patient was given heparin during hospitalization for a deep vein thrombophlebitis of the right lower extremity. The patient had back pain and the nurse was not answering the bell, so he decided to take two aspirin. The interaction between the aspirin and heparin caused a subcutaneous hemorrhage of the thigh of the right lower extremity. How should the interaction between aspirin and heparin coded?

    a. Poisoning codes for aspirin and heparin, and subcutaneous hemorrhage of the thigh of the right lower extremity as secondary conditions

    b. Poisoning codes for aspirin and heparin, and subcutaneous hemorrhage of the thigh of the right lower extremity as principal

    c. Adverse effects of drugs for aspirin and heparin, and subcutaneous hemorrhage of the thigh of the right lower extremity as secondary conditions

    d. Adverse effects of drugs for aspirin and heparin as secondary diagnoses, and subcutaneous hemorrhage of the thigh of the right lower extremity as principal

14. A patient is admitted to the hospital for pain due to pacemaker electrode. The patient also has hypothyroidism due to partial thyroidectomy seven years ago and a breast cyst. The pacemaker electrode was relocated and synthroid was given during hospitalization. The diagnostic codes (excluding E codes) that should be assigned are:

996.0	Mechanical complication of cardiac device, implant, and graft	
996.01	due to cardiac pacemaker (electrode)	
996.6	Infection and inflammatory reaction due to internal prosthetic device, implant and graft	
996.61	due to cardiac device, implant, and graft	
996.7	Other complications of internal (biological) (synthetic) prosthetic device, implant, and graft	
996.72	due to other cardiac device, implant, and graft	
610.0	Solitary cyst of breast	
610.4	Mammary duct ectasia	
244.0	Postsurgical hypothyroidism	
244.1	Other postablative hypothyroidism	
244.9	Unspecified hypothyroidism	
V45.79	Other acquired absence of organ	

a. 996.01, 244.0

b. 996.61, 244.0, 610.0

c. 996.72, 244.0

d. 996.72, 244.0, 610.0

15. A patient was admitted to the emergency department for abdominal pain with diarrhea and was diagnosed with infectious gastroenteritis. The patient also had angina and chronic obstructive pulmonary disease. List the diagnoses that would be coded in the order of sequence.

a. Abdominal pain, infectious gastroenteritis, chronic obstructive pulmonary disease, angina

b. Infectious gastroenteritis, chronic obstructive pulmonary disease, angina

c. Gastroenteritis, abdominal pain, angina

d. Diarrhea, chronic obstructive pulmonary disease, angina

16. A patient was admitted to the endoscopy unit for a screening colonoscopy. During the colonoscopy, polyps of the colon were found and a polypectomy was performed. What diagnostic codes should be used and how should they be sequenced?

V76	Special screening for malignant neoplasms
V76.51	Colon
211	Benign neoplasm of other parts of digestive system
211.3	Benign neoplasm of colon

a. V76.51

b. 211.3

c. V76.51, 211.3

d. 211.3, V76.51

Please refer to the following when answering questions 17 and 18.

216	Benign neoplasm of skin
Includes:	Blue nevus
	dermatofibroma
	hydrocystoma
	pigmented nevus
	syringoadenoma
	syringoma
Excludes:	
	Skin of genital organs (221.0–222.9)

17. When coding benign neoplasm of the skin, the section noted above directs the coder to:

    a. Use category 216 for a syringoma

    b. Use category 216 for malignant melanoma

    c. Use category 216 for malignant neoplasm of the bone

    d. Use category 216 for malignant neoplasm of the skin

18. When coding benign neoplasm of the skin of the labia, the section noted above directs the coder to:

    a. Use category 216

    b. Use category 221.0–222.9

    c. Use category 174

    d. Use category 173

19. A patient was discharged from the same-day-surgery unit with the following diagnoses: mature senile cataract, diabetes mellitus, hypertension, and was treated for mild acute renal failure. Which codes are correct?

250.00	Diabetes mellitus without mention of complication, type II or unspecified type, not stated as uncontrolled
250.40	Diabetes with renal manifestations, type II or unspecified type, not stated as uncontrolled
366.1	Senile cataract
366.10	Senile cataract, unspecified
366.17	Total or mature cataract
401.9	Essential Hypertension, unspecified
403.90	Hypertensive chronic kidney disease, unspecified, with chronic kidney disease stage I through stage IV, or unspecified
584.9	Acute kidney failure, unspecified

    a. 366.10, 250.40, 403.90, 584.9

    b. 366.17, 250.00, 401.9, 584.9

    c. 366.17, 250.40, 403.90, 584.9

    d. 366.10, 250.00, 401.9, 584.9

20. A patient is admitted with an acute exacerbation of COPD with stage V hypertensive kidney disease. What is the correct diagnostic code assignment?

403.90	Hypertensive chronic kidney disease, unspecified, with chronic kidney disease stage I through stage IV or unspecified
403.91	Hypertensive chronic kidney disease, unspecified with, chronic kidney disease stage V or end-stage renal disease
491.21	Obstructive chronic bronchitis, with (acute) exacerbation
496	Chronic airway obstruction, not elsewhere classified
585.5	Chronic kidney disease, stage V

   a. 496, 403.90

   b. 491.21, 403.90

   c. 496, 403.91

   d. 491.21, 403.91, 585.5

21. A patient is admitted with acute respiratory failure, hypertension, and congestive heart failure. The patient was intubated upon admission to the hospital. What are the correct diagnosis codes and sequencing?

401.9	Essential hypertension, unspecified
428.0	Congestive heart failure, unspecified
518.81	Acute respiratory failure
518.82	Other pulmonary insufficiency, NEC
518.83	Chronic respiratory failure
518.84	Acute and chronic respiratory failure
518.89	Other disease of lung, NEC

   a. 518.81, 401.9, 428.0

   b. 428.0, 518.81, 401.9

   c. 518.84, 401.9, 428.0

   d. 428.0, 518.84, 401.9

22. A patient is treated for esophageal varices with hemorrhage due to cirrhosis. The diagnostic codes that would be assigned are:

456.0	Esophageal varices with bleeding
456.1	Esophageal varices without mention of bleeding
456.20	Esophageal varices in diseases classified elsewhere with bleeding
456.21	Esophageal varices in diseases classified elsewhere without mention of bleeding
571.5	Cirrhosis of the liver without mention of alcohol

   a. 456.0, 571.5

   b. 456.20, 571.5

   c. 571.5, 456.0

   d. 571.5, 456.20

23. A patient had a normal pregnancy and delivery with loose nuchal cord around neck. Delivery was accompanied by an episiotomy with birth of liveborn male infant. Delivery room record states "no evidence of fetal problem." What diagnostic and procedure codes should be assigned?

650	Normal delivery
663.11	Cord around neck, with compression, delivered with or without mention of antepartum condition
663.12	Cord around neck, with compression, delivered with mention of postpartum condition
663.31	Other and unspecified cord entanglement, without mention of compression, delivered with or without mention of antepartum condition
663.32	Other and unspecified cord entanglement, without mention of compression, delivered with mention of postpartum condition
V27.0	Single liveborn
73.59	Other manually assisted delivery
73.6	Episiotomy

   a. 650, V27.0, 73.6

   b. 663.31, V27.0, 73.6

   c. 663.31, 73.6

   d. 663.31, V27.0, 73.59

24. Normal twin delivery at 30 weeks. Both babies were delivered vaginally and were liveborn. What conditions should have codes assigned?

644.21	Early onset of delivery, delivered with or without mention of antepartum condition
650	Normal delivery
651.01	Twin pregnancy, delivered with or without mention of antepartum condition
V27.0	Single liveborn
V27.2	Twins, both liveborn

   a. 650, V27.0

   b. 644.21, V27.2

   c. 651.01, 644.21, V27.2

   d. 650, 651.01, V27.2

25. A 45-year-old female with chronic ulcerative enterocolitis and steroid induced osteoporosis due to long-term steroid therapy. What codes should be assigned?

556.0	Ulcerative (chronic) enterocolitis
556.1	Ulcerative (chronic) ileocolitis
733.00	Osteoporosis, unspecified
733.09	Osteoporosis, drug-induced
E932.0	Adverse effects of steroids
V58.65	Long-term (current) use of steroids
V58.69	Long-term (current) use of other medications

   a. 556.0, 733.09, E932.0 V58.65

   b. 556.1, 733.00, E932.0, V58.69

   c. 556.0, 733.00, E932.0 V58.69

   d. 556.1, 733.09, E932.0, V58.65

26. A patient was treated in the emergency department with lacerations of the neck and underwent a repair of two (2) wounds of the neck (2.0 cm and 1.4 cm) with layered closure. What are the diagnostic (excluding E codes) and procedure codes assigned?

874.8	Open wound of neck, Other and unspecified parts, without mention of complication
874.9	Open wound of neck, Other and unspecified parts, with complicated
86.59	Closure of skin and subcutaneous tissue of other sites
12041	Repair, intermediate, wounds of neck, hands, feet and/or external genitalia; 2. 5 cm or less
12042	Repair, intermediate, wounds of neck, hands, feet, and/or external genitalia, 2.6 cm to 7.5 cm

   a. 874.8, 86.59

   b. 874.9, 86.59

   c. 874.8, 12041

   d. 874.8, 12042

27. A 12-year-old boy was seen in an ambulatory surgical center for pain in his right arm. The x-ray showed fracture of ulna. Patient underwent closed reduction of fracture right proximal ulna. What diagnostic and procedure codes should be assigned?

813	Fracture of radius and ulna
813.04	Other and unspecified fractures of proximal end of ulna (alone)
79.02	Closed reduction of fracture without internal fixation; radius and ulna
25560	Closed treatment of radial and ulnar shaft fracture, without manipulation
24670	Closed treatment of ulnar fracture, proximal end (eg, olecranon or coronoid process(es)); without manipulation
24675	Closed treatment of ulnar fracture, proximal end (eg, olecranon or coronoid process(es)); with manipulation

   a. 813, 79.02

   b. 813.04, 79.02

   c. 813.04, 25560

   d. 813.04, 24675

28. Assign the code(s) for endoscopic sinusotomy with bilateral anterior ethmoidectomy.

31231	Nasal endoscopy, diagnostic, unilateral or bilateral (separate procedure)
31254	Nasal/sinus endoscopy, surgical; with ethmoidectomy, partial (anterior)
−50	Bilateral procedure

   a. 31254

   b. 31254–50

   c. 31254, 31254

   d. 31231

29. Assign the code(s) for bronchoscopy with bilateral transbronchial biopsy.

31628	Bronchoscopy, rigid or flexible, including fluoroscopic guidance, when performed; with transbronchial lung biopsy(s), single lobe
31629	Bronchoscopy, rigid or flexible, including fluoroscopic guidance, when performed; with transbronchial needle aspiration biopsy(s), trachea, main stem and/or lobar bronchus(i)
31632	Bronchoscopy, rigid or flexible, including fluoroscopic guidance, when performed; with transbronchial lung biopsy(s), each additional lobe

a. 31628

b. 31628–50

c. 31628, 31632

d. 31629

30. Assign the code(s) for diagnostic left and right cardiac catheterization, left ventriculogram, coronary arteriogram.

37.21	Right heart cardiac catheterization
37.22	Left heart cardiac catheterization
37.23	Combined right and left heart cardiac catheterization
88.53	Angiocardiography of left heart structures
88.54	Combined right and left heart angiocardiography
88.55	Coronary arteriography using a single catheter
88.56	Coronary arteriography using two catheters
88.57	Other and unspecified coronary arteriography

a. 37.21, 37.22, 88.53, 88.55

b. 37.23, 88.57, 88.53

c. 37.23

d. 88.53, 88.55, 37.23

31. Assign the code for dilatation and curettage for missed abortion at 11 weeks' gestation.

69.01	Dilation and curettage for termination of pregnancy
69.02	Dilation and curettage following delivery or abortion
69.09	Other dilation and curettage
69.51	Aspiration curettage of uterus for termination of pregnancy

a. 69.02

b. 69.01

c. 69.09

d. 69.51

32. Assign the code(s) for bilateral epidural lumbar injection of steroids:

62282	Injection/infusion of neurolytic substance (eg, alcohol, phenol, iced saline solutions) with or without other therapeutic substance; epidural, lumbar, sacral (caudal)
62311	Injection(s) of diagnostic or therapeutic substance(s) (including anesthetic, antispasmodic, opioid, steroid, other solution), not including neurolytic substances, including needle or catheter placement, includes contrast for localization when performed, epidural or subarachnoid; lumbar or sacral (caudal)
−50	Bilateral procedure

   a. 62282

   b. 62311

   c. 62311, 62311

   d. 62311–50

33. Assign the code(s) for extraction of extracapsular cataract with simultaneous intraocular lens insertion in the right eye.

66982	Extracapsular cataract removal with insertion of intraocular lens prosthesis (1-stage procedure), manual or mechanical technique (eg, irrigation and aspiration or phacoemulsification), complex requiring devices or techniques not generally used in routine cataract surgery (eg, iris expansion device, suture support for intraocular lens, or primary posterior capsulorhexis), or performed on patients in the amblyogenic developmental stage
66983	Intracapsular cataract extraction with insertion of intraocular lens prosthesis (1-stage procedure)
66984	Extracapsular cataract removal with insertion of intraocular lens prosthesis (1-stage procedure), manual or mechanical technique (eg, irrigation and aspiration or phacoemulsification)
−51	Multiple procedures
−RT	Right side

   a. 66982–RT

   b. 66983–RT

   c. 66984–RT

   d. 66984–51

34. Assign the code(s) for chemotherapy for 3 hours' infusion.

96401	Chemotherapy administration, subcutaneous or intramuscular; non-hormonal anti-neoplastic
96413	Chemotherapy administration, intravenous infusion technique; up to 1 hour, single or initial substance/drug
+96415	each additional hour (List separately in addition to code for primary procedure.)
−51	Multiple procedures

   a. 96413, 96415, 96415

   b. 96413, 96415–51

   c. 96413, 96413, 96413

   d. 96401

35. Assign the code(s) for chest x-ray, complete.

71010	Radiologic examination, chest; single view, frontal
71020	Radiologic examination, chest, 2 views, frontal and lateral
71030	Radiologic examination, chest, complete, minimum 4 views
71035	Radiologic examination, chest, special views (eg, lateral decubitus, Bucky studies)

   a. 71020

   b. 71030

   c. 71010, 71035

   d. 71035

36. Assign the code(s) for mammographic guidance for breast needle localization placement with fine needle aspiration.

77031	Stereotactic localization guidance for breast biopsy or needle placement (eg, for wire localization or for injection), each lesion, radiological supervision and interpretation
77032	Mammographic guidance for needle placement, breast (eg, for wire localization or for injection), each lesion, radiological supervision and interpretation
10021	Fine needle aspiration, without imaging guidance
10022	Fine needle aspiration, with imaging guidance

   a. 77032

   b. 10022

   c. 77032, 10022

   d. 77031

37. A laparoscopic tubal ligation is completed. What is the correct CPT code assignment?

49320	Laparoscopy, abdomen, peritoneum, and omentum, diagnostic, with or without collection of specimen(s) by brushing or washing (separate procedure)
58662	Laparoscopy, surgical; with fulguration or excision of lesions of the ovary, pelvic viscera, or peritoneal surface by any method
58670	Laparoscopy, surgical; with fulguration of oviducts (with or without transection)
58671	Laparoscopy, surgical; with occlusion of oviducts by device (eg, band, clip, or Falope ring)

   a. 49320, 58662

   b. 58670

   c. 58671

   d. 49320

38. A laparoscopic cholecystectomy was performed. What is the correct ICD-9-CM procedure code?

51.21	Other partial cholecystectomy
51.22	Cholecystectomy
51.23	Laparoscopic cholecystectomy
51.24	Laparoscopic partial cholecystectomy

a. 51.21

b. 51.22

c. 51.23

d. 51.24

Domain III **Regulatory Guidelines and Reporting Requirements for Acute-Care (Inpatient) Service**

39. Hospital A: The patient is admitted for chest pain and is found to have an acute inferior myocardial infarction with atrial fibrillation. After the atrial fibrillation was controlled and the patient was stabilized, the patient was transferred to Hospital B for a CABG X3. The appropriate sequencing and ICD codes for both hospitalizations would be:

414.01	Coronary atherosclerosis of native coronary artery
410.41	Acute myocardial infarction of other inferior wall, initial episode of care
410.42	Acute myocardial infarction of other inferior wall, subsequent episode of care
410.91	Acute myocardial infarction of unspecified site, initial episode of care
410.92	Acute myocardial infarction of unspecified site, subsequent episode of care
427.31	Atrial fibrillation
786.50	Chest pain, unspecified
36.13	Aortocoronary bypass of three coronary arteries

a. Hospital A: 786.50, 410.91, 427.31: Hospital B: 410.92, 427.31, 36.13

b. Hospital A: 410.41, 427.31: Hospital B: 410.92, 427.31, 36.13

c. Hospital A: 410.41, 427.31: Hospital B: 414.01, 410.41, 427.31, 36.13

d. Hospital A: 410.42, 427.31: Hospital B: 410.41, 427.31, 36.13

40. A patient is admitted and discharged with chest pain. After evaluation, it is suspected the patient may have gastroesophageal reflux disease (GERD). The final diagnosis was "Rule out GERD." The correct code assignment would be:

a. V71.7, Observation for suspected cardiovascular disease

b. 789.01, Abdominal pain, right upper quadrant

c. 530.81, Esophageal reflux

d. 786.50, Chest pain, unspecified

41. If a patient has a principal diagnosis of septicemia, which of the following procedures will increase the DRG assignment the most?

a. Bronchoscopy with biopsy (33.24)

b. Debridement of nails (86.27)

c. Nonexcisional debridement of skin ulcer with abrasion (86.28)

d. Ventilator management for 106 consecutive hours (96.72)

42. A patient presents to a facility with a history of prostate cancer and mental confusion on admission. The patient completed radiation therapy for prostatic carcinoma three years ago and is status post a radical resection of the prostate. A CT scan of the brain reveals metastatic carcinoma of the brain. The correct coding and sequencing of this patient's record is:

a. Metastatic carcinoma of the brain, carcinoma of the prostate, mental confusion

b. Mental confusion, history of carcinoma of the prostate, admission for chemotherapy

c. Metastatic carcinoma of the brain, history of carcinoma of the prostate

d. Carcinoma of the prostate, metastatic carcinoma to the brain

43. The patient is discharged with hemiplegia and aphasia associated with a cerebral infarction of the left side of the brain. The patient is right-handed and also has a history of hypertension and compensated congestive heart failure (both conditions currently controlled on medication and treated while in the hospital). What code assignment would be appropriate?

342.90	Hemiplegia, unspecified, affecting unspecified side
342.91	Hemiplegia, unspecified, affecting dominant side
342.92	Hemiplegia, unspecified, affecting nondominant side
434.90	Cerebral artery occlusion unspecified, without mention of cerebral infarction
434.91	Cerebral artery occlusion unspecified, with cerebral infarction
401.9	Essential hypertension, unspecified
428.0	Congestive heart failure, unspecified
784.3	Aphasia

a. 434.91, 342.91, 784.3, 428.0, 401.9

b. 342.90, 784.3, 428.0, 401.9

c. 434.90, 342.90, 784.3

d. 434.91, 342.90, 784.3

44. A patient is admitted with hemoptysis. A bronchoscopy with transbronchial biopsy of the lower lobe was undertaken that revealed squamous cell carcinoma of the lung. Which conditions should be identified as present on admission?

770.3	Pulmonary hemorrhage
786.30	Hemoptysis, unspecified
162.5	Malignant neoplasm of lower lobe, bronchus or lung

a. 162.5

b. 786.2, 786.30

c. 162.5, 786.30

d. 162.5, 770.3, 786.30

45. Medicare reimbursement depends on the following, *except*:

   a. The correct designation of the principal diagnosis

   b. Policies and procedures of the medical staff

   c. The presence or absence of additional codes that represent complications, comorbidities, or major complications/comorbidities

   d. Procedures performed

46. A coder reviews a medical record and determines that a code Medicare has designated as "unacceptable principal diagnosis" is the correct code to assign. What should the coder do?

   a. Assign a code from the history and physician as the principal diagnosis

   b. Assign the code even though the insurer may not pay the claim

   c. Use a comorbidity as the principal diagnosis

   d. Assign a code from the outpatient visit prior to admission

47. A condition is present on admission when:

   a. It is the principal diagnosis

   b. It is accordance with medical staff bylaws

   c. A condition that occurs prior to an inpatient admission

   d. It is present within 3 days after admission

48. Documentation from the nursing or other allied health professionals' notes can be used to establish which of the following diagnoses:

   a. Body mass index (BMI)

   b. Malnutrition

   c. Aspiration pneumonia

   d. Fatigue

Domain IV *Regulatory Guidelines and Reporting Requirements for Outpatient Services*

49. Carcinoma of multiple overlapping sites of the bladder. Diagnostic cystoscopy and transurethral fulguration of bladder lesions (1.9 cm, 6.0 cm) are completed and a skin lesion was also removed from the left thigh. What modifier should be added to the procedure codes?

   a. −50, Bilateral procedure

   b. −51, Multiple procedures

   c. −59, Distinct procedure service

   d. −99, Multiple modifiers

50. A bronchoscopy with biopsy of the left bronchus was completed and revealed adenocarcinoma. What, if any, modifier should be added to the procedure codes?

    a. −50, Bilateral procedure

    b. −51, Multiple procedures

    c. −59, Distinct procedure service

    d. No modifiers should be reported.

51. Wide excision of 0.65-cm malignant melanoma (margins included) from right forearm. The diagnosis and procedure codes reported are:

172.6	Malignant melanoma of skin; upper limb, including shoulder
195.4	Malignant neoplasm of upper limb
11401	Excision, benign lesion including margins, except skin tag (unless listed elsewhere), trunk, arms, or legs; excised diameter 0.6 to 1.0 cm
11601	Excision, malignant lesion including margins, trunk, arms, or legs; excised diameter 0.6 to 1.0 cm
25075	Excision, tumor, soft tissue of forearm and/or wrist area; subcutaneous, less than 3 cm

    a. 172.6, 11401

    b. 195.4, 11601

    c. 172.6, 11601

    d. 172.6, 25705

52. What diagnoses and procedures should be reported for colonoscopy with cauterization of diverticular bleeding?

578.9	Hemorrhage of gastrointestinal tract, unspecified
562.10	Diverticulosis of colon (without mention of hemorrhage)
562.12	Diverticulosis of colon with hemorrhage
563.13	Diverticulitis of colon with hemorrhage
45378	Colonoscopy, flexible, proximal to splenic flexure, diagnostic, with or without collection of specimen(s) by brushing or washing, with or without colon decompression (separate procedure)
45382	Colonoscopy, flexible, proximal to splenic flexure; with control of bleeding (eg, injection, bipolar cautery, unipolar cautery, laser, heater probe, stapler, plasma, coagulator)

    a. 562.10, 578.9, 45382

    b. 562.12, 45382

    c. 563.13, 45382

    d. 578.9, 562.10, 45382

53. What diagnoses and procedures should be reported for recurrent left inguinal hernia with laparoscopic repair?

550.91	Inguinal hernia, without mention of obstruction or gangrene, unilateral or unspecified, recurrent
550.10	Inguinal hernia, with obstruction, without mention of gangrene, unilateral or unspecified (not specified as recurrent)
550.11	Inguinal hernia, with obstruction, without mention of gangrene, unilateral or unspecified, recurrent
49520	Repair recurrent inguinal hernia, any age, reducible
49521	Repair recurrent inguinal hernia, any age, reducible, incarcerated or strangulated
49651	Laparoscopy, surgical, repair recurrent inguinal hernia

   a. 550.91, 49520

   b. 550.11, 49521

   c. 550.91, 49651

   d. 550.10, 49520

54. A patient was admitted after a fall down the steps. The patient was unconscious for approximately 45 minutes and was admitted to the emergency department (ED) within 3 hours of the fall. A CT scan was performed within an hour of admission to the ED. A skull vault fracture with cerebral contusion was diagnosed by the ED physician based on the findings in the CT scan. What conditions should be reported on the Unified Billing form 04 (UB-04)?

780.09	Alterations of consciousness; other (drowsiness, semicoma, unconsciousness, somnolence, stupor)
800.12	Fracture of vault of skull, closed with cerebral laceration and contusion, with brief (less than 1 hour) loss of consciousness
803.12	Other and unqualified skull fractures, closed with cerebral laceration and contusion, with brief (less than 1 hour) loss of consciousness
803.42	Other and unqualified skull fractures, closed with intracranial injury of other and unspecified nature, with brief (less than 1 hour) loss of consciousness
851.82	Other and unspecified cerebral laceration and contusion, without mentioning of open intracranial wound, with brief (less than 1 hour) loss of consciousness
V71.4	Observation following other accident
E880.9	Fall on or from stairs or steps; other stairs or steps

   a. 800.12, E880.9

   b. 780.09

   c. 803.02, E880.9

   d. 800.12, E880.9

55. The UHDDS definition of principal diagnosis does not apply to the coding of outpatient encounters because:

   a. There is not enough documentation

   b. Usually there are multiple reasons for the encounter

   c. No after study element is involved as continued evaluation cannot occur

   d. A pre-admission work up is not available

56. Coding professionals need to have surgical references in order to discriminate between:

    a. Correct and incorrect documentation based on Joint Commission requirements

    b. Reportable and nonreportable procedures

    c. Chemotherapeutic drugs

    d. A comorbid condition and a complication that prolongs the length of stay

57. In 2000 the Centers for Medicare and Medicaid Services (CMS) issued the final rule on the outpatient prospective payment system (OPPS). This program:

    a. Identified the payment structure for long-term care

    b. Divided outpatient services into fixed-payment groups

    c. Created less opportunity for health information management professionals

    d. Facilitated greater use of ICD-9-CM procedure codes

58. The use of the outpatient code editor (OCE) is designed to:

    a. Correct documentation of home health visits

    b. Facilitate reporting of adverse drug events

    c. Reduce the use of computer assisted coding

    d. Identify incomplete or incorrect claims

Domain V   *Data Quality and Management*

59. A 64-year-old female was discharged with the final diagnosis of acute renal failure and hypertension. What coding rule applies?

    a. Use combination code of hypertension and renal failure.

    b. Use separate codes for hypertension and chronic renal failure.

    c. Use separate codes for hypertension and acute renal failure.

    d. Use separate codes for elevated blood pressure and chronic renal failure.

60. Cystourethroscopy with removal of two lesions of separate locations in the bladder, one is 1.5-cm bladder tumor anterior wall and one is 0.75-cm in the lateral wall. What coding rule applies?

    a. Two CPT codes should be used with a modifier −59.

    b. Two CPT codes should be used.

    c. Code only the CPT code for cystourethroscopy.

    d. Code only the largest tumor.

61. Diagnostic-related groups (DRGs) and ambulatory patient classifications (APCs) are similar in that they are both:

    a. Determined by HCPCS codes

    b. Focused on hospital outpatients

    c. Focused on hospital inpatients

    d. Prospective payment systems

Please refer to the following data when answering questions 62 and 63 (Note: The DRG numbers and weights are not actual numbers and weights for fiscal year 2013.)

MS-DRG	MS-DRG Wt.	Number of Patients
191	2.0	10
192	1.5	10
193	1.0	10

62. The case-mix index for the information provided above is:

    a. 0.679

    b. 0.89

    c. 1.5

    d. 0.75

63. The information provided shows that:

    a. The payment is higher for patients with DRG 191

    b. There are more patients with DRG 191

    c. The case-mix index could be increased if more patients in DRG 193 were admitted

    d. The case mix would not increase if more patients in DRG 193 were admitted

64. Generally, data quality is defined as:

    a. Ensuring the greatest amount of data possible is obtained from the medical record

    b. Ensuring the accuracy and completeness of an organization's data

    c. Ensuring accuracy of the case-mix index

    d. Ensuring the optimal reimbursement for each encounter

65. A method of checking the accuracy of data is to:

    a. Validate the purpose for the data collection

    b. Warehouse data on a regular basis

    c. Authenticate all end users

    d. Ensure that each record or entry within the database is correct

66. When applying AHIMA's 10 data characteristics to a patient encounter, a data quality checkpoint for data timeliness during medication reconciliation would be:

    a. Patient's medications are available for patient care

    b. Ensuring a standardized formulary

    c. Attributes for each medication are defined

    d. Checks are done to ensure that what is ordered is what is given to the patient

67. Before an organization can measure the quality of information it produces it must:

   a. Establish a data quality committee

   b. Investigate if there are fraudulent processes in current use

   c. Determine all attributes of poor quality

   d. Establish data standards within the organization

Domain VI | *Information and Communication Technologies*

68. A surgeon would like to undertake a research study on his patients with stage II malignant melanoma of the back, who have undergone wide excision of the melanoma. What work processes and associated software could be used to provide this information?

   a. Obtain a summary of the cases from the cancer registry, import them into a spreadsheet, and provide to the surgeon.

   b. Obtain a summary of the cases from the chart completion software, import them into a spreadsheet, and provide to the surgeon.

   c. Obtain a summary of the cases from the master patient index, import them into a spreadsheet, and provide to the surgeon.

   d. Obtain a summary of the cases from the transcription tracking software, import them into a spreadsheet, and provide to the surgeon.

69. The coding supervisor is concerned that patients diagnosed with carcinoid colon tumors were miscoded as malignant during the last six months. To address this situation, what work processes could be undertaken?

   a. Obtain the cases of carcinoid colon tumors from the cancer registry, obtain the cases of malignant colon tumors from the billing system, import both lists into a spreadsheet, and compare them. The cases in the cancer registry and not in the billing system are likely malignant and should be manually reviewed.

   b. Compare the cases from the chart completion software with the billing software. Identify the cases that are not in the billing system. These cases should be manually reviewed to ensure they are not carcinoid tumors.

   c. Obtain the cases of malignant colon tumors from both the cancer registry and the billing system; import both lists into a spreadsheet and compare them. Identify the cases that are not in the tumor registry that are in the billing system. These cases should be manually reviewed to ensure they are not carcinoid tumors.

   d. Compare the cases from the transcription tracking software to the billing system. Identify the cases that are not in the transcription tracking software and are in the billing system. These cases should be manually reviewed to ensure they are not carcinoid tumors.

70. A quality improvement study showed that newborn codes associated with maternal conditions are not being coded as often as they should. What HIM software could be used to identify the mother's chart so it can be reviewed at the time the newborn record is coded?

   a. Birth certificate registry or master patient index

   b. Transcription registry or correspondence registry

   c. Quality improvement or operative registry

   d. Pathology or laboratory information

71. An entity relationship diagram was developed to depict:

    a. How departments within the organization relate to each other

    b. Timeframes for fiscal intermediary payment distribution

    c. Reporting structures of the medical staff

    d. Relational database structures

72. A data map or crosswalk consists of:

    a. Terms used to describe paths between classifications and vocabularies

    b. A map of time frames for multiple project completion

    c. A descriptive list of data names

    d. Normalized data attributes

73. An object-oriented database contains:

    a. A database administrator

    b. A description of register elements

    c. Data and their relationships within a single structure

    d. Distributed data requirements

74. The most common language used for both data definition language and data manipulation language is:

    a. Unified modeling language

    b. JAVA

    c. Perl

    d. Structured query language

Domain VII *Privacy, Confidentiality, Legal, and Ethical Issues*

75. A facility located near a national park has a significant number of snake bites, and patients receive treatment with antivenom in urgent-care settings. Sometimes a patient is admitted to the hospital after several days. Can the urgent-care setting provide the hospital with a list of names of patients treated with snake antivenom?

    a. Only the names of patients who are admitted to the hospital can be requested if the physician needs it for continuity of care, but an entire list of patients cannot be provided.

    b. A list of names could be provided.

    c. No information can be obtained under any circumstances.

    d. A list of patients may be available after consultation with the national park ranger.

76. When patients are admitted with vaginal bleeding, one of the financial analysts has determined that if one additional procedure code were routinely added to each case, reimbursement would be increased. This would be considered an ethical practice if:

    a. The vice president of finance approves the procedure

    b. The billing department wants this; it can be done

    c. Under no circumstances could this be done

    d. There is documentation of the procedure in the medical record

77. The patient was admitted for breast carcinoma in the right breast at two o'clock. This was removed via lumpectomy. The patient was found to have 1 of 7 lymph nodes positive for carcinoma during axillary lymph node dissection. One of the patient's neighbors who is also a coworker at the hospital called the coding department to get the patient's diagnosis because she is a cancer survivor herself. The coder should:

    a. Discuss the case with the coworker

    b. Report the incident to hospital security

    c. Give the caller false information

    d. Explain that discussing the case would violate the patient's right to privacy

78. The billing department has requested that copies of the final coding summary with associated code meanings for Medicare be printed remotely in the admission department. Currently they request the summaries only when there is an unspecified procedure. Each time the coding supervisor goes to the admission department, the coding summaries have been left on a table near the patient entrance. Of the actions presented here, what would be the best action for the coding supervisor to take?

    a. Comply with the request.

    b. Refuse to undertake this without further explanation.

    c. Ignore the request.

    d. Explain to the billing department supervisor that leaving the coding summary in public view violates the patient's right to privacy.

79. Inpatients who undergo open reduction and internal fixation of a fractured femur are routinely coded with blood loss anemia because of a policy that specifies that this should be done when there is intraoperative blood loss of 500 cc or more documented in the operative report and the patient has a low hemoglobin. Why is this correct or incorrect?

    a. It is correct to code blood loss anemia because the policy requires it.

    b. It is correct because the clinical signs are documented in the record.

    c. It is incorrect because the patient must also have a blood transfusion in order for blood loss anemia to be coded.

    d. It is incorrect because the physician did not document the blood loss anemia in the progress notes.

80. A female patient is admitted for a second-degree cystocele. A repair is performed. In order to code this accurately, what document provides the required additional information?

    a. History and physical

    b. Discharge summary

    c. Consultation

    d. Operative report

81. In order to accurately code a cardiac catheterization, what needs to be determined based on a review of the documentation?

    a. The approach and the side of the heart (chambers) into which the catheter was inserted

    b. The approach, the side of the heart (chambers) into which the catheter was inserted, as well as any additional procedures performed

    c. The duration of the procedure

    d. If there is documentation of the procedure in the medical record that stents are considered

Multiple Select Questions

Use the following list of codes and select all answers that apply for the following multiple select questions.

401.0	Essential hypertension, malignant
401.1	Essential hypertension, benign
401.9	Essential hypertension, unspecified
402.00	Hypertensive heart disease, malignant, without heart failure
402.01	Hypertensive heart disease, malignant, with heart failure
402.10	Hypertensive heart disease, benign without heart failure
402.11	Hypertensive heart disease, benign with heart failure
402.90	Hypertensive heart disease, unspecified without heart failure
402.91	Hypertensive heart disease, unspecified with heart failure
403.00	Hypertensive chronic kidney disease, malignant, with chronic kidney disease stage I through IV or unspecified
403.01	Hypertensive chronic kidney disease, malignant, with chronic kidney disease stage V or end-stage
403.10	Hypertensive chronic kidney disease, benign, with chronic kidney disease stage I through IV or unspecified
403.11	Hypertensive chronic kidney disease, benign, with chronic kidney disease stage I through V or end-stage
403.90	Hypertensive chronic kidney disease, unspecified, with chronic kidney disease stage I through IV or unspecified
403.91	Hypertensive chronic kidney disease, unspecified, with chronic kidney disease stage V or end-stage
404.00	Hypertensive heart and chronic kidney disease, malignant, without heart failure and with chronic kidney disease stage I through IV or unspecified
404.01	Hypertensive heart and chronic kidney disease, malignant, with heart failure and with chronic kidney disease stage I through IV or unspecified
404.02	Hypertensive heart and chronic kidney disease, malignant, without heart failure and with chronic kidney disease stage V or end-stage
404.03	Hypertensive heart and chronic kidney disease, malignant, with heart failure and with chronic kidney disease stage V or end-stage
404.10	Hypertensive heart and chronic kidney disease, benign, without heart failure and with chronic kidney disease stage I through IV or unspecified
404.11	Hypertensive heart and chronic kidney disease, benign, with heart failure and with chronic kidney disease stage I through IV or unspecified
404.12	Hypertensive heart and chronic kidney disease, benign, without heart failure and with chronic kidney disease stage V through end-stage
404.13	Hypertensive heart and chronic kidney disease, benign with heart failure and with chronic kidney disease stage V through end-stage
404.90	Hypertensive heart and chronic kidney disease, unspecified, without heart failure and with chronic kidney disease stage I through IV or unspecified
404.91	Hypertensive heart and chronic kidney disease, unspecified, with heart failure and with chronic kidney disease stage I through IV or unspecified
404.92	Hypertensive heart and chronic kidney disease, unspecified, without heart failure and with chronic kidney disease stage V through end-stage
404.93	Hypertensive heart and chronic kidney disease, unspecified, with heart failure and with chronic kidney disease stage V through end-stage
405.01	Secondary hypertension, malignant renovascular
405.09	Secondary hypertension, malignant other
405.11	Secondary hypertension, benign renovascular
405.19	Secondary hypertension, benign other
405.91	Secondary hypertension, unspecified, renovascular
405.99	Secondary hypertension, unspecified, other
428.0	Congestive heart failure, unspecified
584. 9	Acute kidney failure, unspecified
585.1	Chronic kidney disease, stage I
585.2	Chronic kidney disease, stage II (mild)
585.3	Chronic kidney disease, stage III (moderate)
585.4	Chronic kidney disease, stage IV (severe)
585.5	Chronic kidney disease, stage V
585.6	End-stage renal disease
585.9	Chronic kidney disease, unspecified
586	Renal failure, unspecified

82. A 77-year-old patient has hypertensive heart disease with congestive heart failure and stage V renal disease. What codes would be assigned? (Select all that apply.)

    a. 402.91, Hypertensive heart disease, unspecified with heart failure

    b. 404.93, Hypertensive heart and chronic kidney disease, unspecified with heart failure and with chronic kidney disease stage V through end-stage

    c. 428.0, Congestive heart failure, unspecified

    d. 585.6, End-stage renal disease

    e. 405.91, Secondary hypertension, unspecified

    f. 585.5, Chronic kidney disease, stage V

83. A 70-year-old patient has congestive heart failure and hypertension with end-stage renal disease. What codes would be assigned? (Select all that apply.)

    a. 402.91, Hypertensive heart disease, unspecified with heart failure

    b. 404.93, Hypertensive heart and chronic kidney disease, unspecified with heart failure and chronic kidney disease stage V through end-stage

    c. 428.0, Congestive heart failure, unspecified

    d. 585.6, End-stage renal disease

    e. 403.91, Hypertensive chronic kidney disease, unspecified with chronic kidney disease stage V or end-stage

    f. 585.5, Chronic kidney disease, stage V

84. A 35-year-old woman has hypertension with acute renal failure and stage III chronic kidney disease. What codes would be assigned? (Select all that apply.)

    a. 584.9, Acute kidney failure, unspecified

    b. 404.93, Hypertensive heart and chronic kidney disease, unspecified with heart failure and chronic kidney disease stage V through end stage

    c. 428.0, Congestive heart failure, unspecified

    d. 403.90, Hypertensive chronic kidney disease, unspecified with chronic kidney disease stage I through IV or unspecified

    e. 401.9, Essential hypertension, unspecified

    f. 585.3, Chronic kidney disease, stage III (moderate)

85. A 55 year patient has malignant hypertensive heart disease with congestive heart failure. What codes would be assigned? (Select all that apply.)

    a. 402.91, Hypertensive heart disease, unspecified with heart failure

    b. 402.01, Hypertensive heart disease, malignant with heart failure

    c. 428.0, Congestive heart failure, unspecified

    d. 585.6, End-stage renal disease

    e. 405.91, Secondary hypertension, unspecified

    f. 585.5, Chronic kidney disease, stage V

86. The CPT definition of a *surgical package* contains which of the following? (Select all that apply.)

    a. The surgical procedure(s)

    b. Local infiltration, metacarpal/metatarsal/digital block, or topical anesthesia

    c. Preoperative tests

    d. Yearly follow-up visits

    e. Typical postoperative follow-up care

    f. Follow-up surgery

87. Current Procedural Terminology (CPT) defines a separate procedure as which of the following? (Select all that apply.)

    a. When performed in conjunction with another service, is considered an integral part of the major service

    b. Provision of anesthesia

    c. Joint aspiration is required

    d. Pre-operative evaluation is not required

    e. E/M codes are needed

    f. The CPT code description includes "separate procedure"

88. Using the following evaluation and management map, which answers represent documentation that should be considered, when assigning an E/M example for hospital acuity points assignment? (Select all that apply.)

Evaluation and Management Mapping

The following are the points needed to determine the level of CPT code:

    Level 1 = 1–20

    Level 2 = 21–35

    Level 3 = 36–47

    Level 4 = 48–60

    Level 5 = > 61

    Critical Care > 61 with constant physician attendance

CPT Codes

Level 1 = 99281	99281–25 with procedure/laboratory/radiology
Level 2 = 99282	99282–25 with procedure/laboratory/radiology
Level 3 = 99283	99283–25 with procedure/laboratory/radiology
Level 4 = 99284	99284–25 with procedure/laboratory/radiology
Level 5 = 99285	99285–25 with procedure/laboratory/radiology

Emergency Department Acuity Points					
	5	10	15	20	25
Meds Given	0–2	3–5	6–7	8–9	> 10
Extent of Hx	Brief	PF	EPF	Detail	Comprehensive
Extent of Exam	Brief	PF	EPF	Detail	Comprehensive
Number of Tests Ordered	0–1	2–3	4–5	6–7	> 8
Supplies Used	1	2–3	4–5	6–7	> 8

a. The surgical procedure performed

b. The anesthesia provided

c. Number of tests ordered

d. The post visit follow-up date

e. Supplies used

f. Medication given

89. To accurately code wound closures, what questions need to be answered? (Select all that apply.)

a. The number of surgical procedures undertaken

b. What type of repair was undertaken: simple, intermediate, or complex?

c. Number of tests ordered

d. The site or body part involved, and what is the extent of the wound?

e. Supplies used

f. What is the length of the repair in centimeters?

1.	24.	47.	70.
2.	25.	48.	71.
3.	26.	49.	72.
4.	27.	50.	73.
5.	28.	51.	74.
6.	29.	52.	75.
7.	30.	53.	76.
8.	31.	54.	77.
9.	32.	55.	78.
10.	33.	56.	79.
11.	34.	57.	80.
12.	35.	58.	81.
13.	36.	59.	82.
14.	37.	60.	83.
15.	38.	61.	84.
16.	39.	62.	85.
17.	40.	63.	86.
18.	41.	64.	87.
19.	42.	65.	88.
20.	43.	66.	89.
21.	44.	67.	
22.	45.	68.	
23.	46.	69.	

CCS

PRACTICE CASE STUDIES

Note: Review the Procedures for Coding Medical Record Cases for the CCS Examination in the Introduction of this book

AMBULATORY CASE—PATIENT 1

FACE SHEET

DATE OF ADMISSION: 4/5   **DATE OF DISCHARGE:** 4/5

SEX: Male   **AGE:** 37   **DISCHARGE DISPOSITION:** Home

ADMISSION DIAGNOSIS: Left inguinal hernia

DISCHARGE DIAGNOSIS: Same

PROCEDURES: Left inguinal herniorrhaphy with excision of lipoma of spermatic cord

HISTORY AND PHYSICAL EXAMINATION—PATIENT 1

ADMITTED: 4/5

HISTORY OF PRESENT ILLNESS: The patient has been well until several months ago when he began to have pain when lifting.

PAST MEDICAL HISTORY: The patient has no other significant medical or surgical history.

SOCIAL HISTORY: Does not use alcohol or tobacco.

ALLERGIES: No known allergies

MEDICATIONS: None

REVIEW OF SYSTEMS:

    SKIN: Warm and dry, mucous membranes moist

    HEENT: Essentially normal

    LUNGS: Clear to percussion and auscultation

    HEART: Normal, regular rhythm

    ABDOMEN: Normal

    GENITALIA: Palpable mass in inguinal canal

    RECTAL: Normal

    EXTREMITIES: No edema

    NEUROLOGIC: Deep tendon reflexes normal

IMPRESSION: Left inguinal hernia

PLAN: Surgical repair of inguinal hernia

PROGRESS NOTES — PATIENT 1

DATE	NOTE
4/5	Nursing:
	Betadine scrub performed, patient anxious to get surgery over; preoperative medications given as ordered.
4/5	Attending MD:
	Brief op note
	Dx: Left inguinal hernia
	Px: Left inguinal herniorrhaphy
	Anes: Local plus sedation
	Complications: None
4/5	Attending MD:
	No bleeding; patient okay for discharge.

OPERATIVE REPORT — PATIENT 1

DATE: 4/5

PREOPERATIVE DIAGNOSIS: Left direct inguinal hernia

POSTOPERATIVE DIAGNOSIS: Left direct inguinal hernia

OPERATION: Left inguinal herniorrhaphy

ANESTHESIA: Local plus sedation

OPERATIVE INDICATIONS: A wide mouth direct sac was present in the lower inguinal canal. A lipoma of the cord was present, but no indirect sac.

OPERATIVE PROCEDURE: Under local anesthesia consisting of the equivalent of 19 cc of 1% Xylocaine and 8 cc of 0.5% Marcaine, the abdomen was prepared with Betadine and sterilely draped. A left inguinal incision was made and carried down through subcutaneous tissues to the aponeurosis of the external oblique, which was opened from the external ring to a point over the internal ring. Flaps were cleaned in both directions. The nerve was retracted inferiorly. The cord structures were separated from the surrounding at the level of the pubic tubercle and retracted with a Penrose drain. Cremaster over the cord was opened and a search made for an indirect sac. None was found. Lipoma of the cord was dissected free and clamped at its base and excised. The base was ligated with 00 chromic catgut. Additional cremasteric muscles were divided and ligated with 00 chromic catgut. The direct sac was further dissected down to its base and inverted as the defect was closed by approximating transversus to transversus with a running suture of 00 Vicryl. The floor of the canal was then closed by approximating the internal oblique to the shelving portion of the inguinal ligament with multiple sutures of 0 Ethibond. The external oblique aponeurosis was then reclosed with 0 Ethibond, leaving the cord and nerve in the subcutaneous position. Several sutures of 0 Ethibond were also placed above the emergence of the cord at the internal ring. Subcutaneous tissues were then approximated with 3-0 Vicryl and after irrigation skin was closed with skin clips. The patient tolerated the procedure well and was sent to the recovery room in good condition.

PATHOLOGY REPORT—PATIENT 1

DATE SPECIMEN SUBMITTED: 4/5

SPECIMEN: Lipoma of cord

CLINICAL DATA:

GROSS DESCRIPTION: The specimen is submitted as lipoma of cord. It consists of a single irregularly shaped fragment of fatty tissue that is 8.0 × 4.0 × 1.5 cm. It is covered with a thin membrane.

MICROSCOPIC DESCRIPTION:

DIAGNOSIS: Lipomatous tissue of left spermatic cord

PHYSICIAN'S ORDERS—PATIENT 1

DATE	ORDER
4/5	Attending MD:
	Admit to same-day surgery
	Betadine scrub ×3 Preop
	May take own meds
4/5	Anesthesia note:
	Continue NPO
	Demerol 50 mg IM 1½ hr Preop
	Vistaril 50 mg IM 1½ hr Preop
	Atropine 0.4 mg IM 1½ hr Preop
4/5	Attending MD:
	Vital signs q. 15 min until stable
	Regular diet
	Darvocet-N-100 q. 4 hrs p.r.n. pain
	Discharge to home when stable

LABORATORY REPORTS—PATIENT 1

HEMATOLOGY

DATE: 4/5

Specimen	Results	Normal Values
WBC	6.83	4.3–11.0
RBC	4.57	4.5–5.9
HGB	13.7	13.5–17.5
HCT	43	41–52
MCV	87.0	80–100
MCHC	35	31–57
PLT	300	150–400

AUTO DIFFERENTIAL—PATIENT 1

DATE: 4/5

Specimen	Results	Normal Values
NEUT	68.3	40.0–74.0
LYMPH	20	19.0–48.0
MONO	5.6	3.4–9.0
EOS	5.6	0.0–7.0
BASO	0.6	0.0–1.5
LUC	3.8	0.0–4.0

URINALYSIS—PATIENT 1

DATE: 4/5

Test	Result	Ref Range
SP GRAVITY	1.017	1.005–1.035
PH	6	5–7
PROT	TRACE	NEG
GLUC	NONE	NEG
KETONES	NONE	NEG
BILI	NONE	NEG
BLOOD	TRACE	NEG
NITRATES	NONE	NEG
RBCS	NONE	NEG
WBCS	NONE	NEG

RADIOLOGY REPORT—PATIENT 1

DATE: 4/5

DIAGNOSIS: Inguinal hernia

EXAMINATION: Chest x-ray

Heart size and shape are acceptable. The lung fields are clear and the pulmonary vascular pattern is unremarkable. There is no free fluid and the trachea remains midline.

Enter two diagnosis codes and two procedure codes.

PDX

DX2

PP1

PR2

AMBULATORY CASE—PATIENT 2

DIAGNOSIS: Low back pain, lumbar radiculopathy with chronic pain syndrome

HISTORY: This is an 18-year-old white female with low back pain and lumbar radicular pain for epidural steroid injection. The patient had an epidural approximately three weeks ago with approximately 30% improvement. The patient is agreeable for an additional epidural steroid injection for pain management.

PROCEDURE: Epidural steroid injection under C-arm guidance via caudal approach and epidurogram. The patient was transferred to the operating room and placed in the prone position. Under MAC anesthesia her low back and sacral areas were sterilely prepped and draped. Local 1% lidocaine was applied with a #23-gauge needle through the skin and surrounding tissues of the sacral hiatus. Then a #17-gauge Epimed needle was inserted percutaneously through the sacral hiatus into the epidural space. This was confirmed via lateral view of the C-arm. Then under AP fluoroscopy, a #18-gauge Epimed catheter was guided to the mid L3-L4 area of the nerve root in the midline. Next, 2 cc of Isovue dye were injected, which showed good bilateral spread in the epidural space. A solution of 6 cc of normal saline, 80 mg of Depo-Medrol and 2 cc of 1% lidocaine was partially deposited at the L3-L4 nerve root. The catheter was then moved down to the L4-L5 nerve root in the midline of the epidural space. An additional 1 cc of Isovue dye was injected, which showed good bilateral spread. An additional one third of local anesthetic Depo-Medrol solution was deposited at the L4-L5 nerve root. The catheter was then moved down to the L5-S1 nerve root and in the midline. Another 1 cc of Isovue dye was injected, which confirmed good bilateral spread and highlighting of the L5-S1 nerve roots bilateral. The remaining local anesthetic Depo-Medrol solution was deposited at the L5-S1 nerve root. The catheter and needle were then pulled intact and the patient was transferred to the recovery room in satisfactory condition.

IMPRESSION: Low back pain, lumbar radiculopathy. This is the patient's second epidural steroid injection.

FOLLOW-UP: After seeing improvement in the next 24 to 48 hours and repeat injection if necessary.

Enter two diagnosis codes and one procedure code.

PDX

DX2

PP1

AMBULATORY RECORD—PATIENT 3

DATE: 8/12/20XX

SURGERY RECORD:

PATIENT HISTORY: This patient is seen today to insert an intrathecal pump for pain management due to ductal carcinoma of the left upper breast metastatic to the spine. She previously underwent modified radical mastectomy with general anesthesia and had no adverse effects. No other surgical history is given. No known allergies, no current medications. Review of systems is normal ASA = 2.

Following preoperative evaluation and discussion with the patient, local anesthesia was used to implant an intrathecal programmable pump surgically placed and attached to a previously placed catheter. The patient tolerated the procedure well. There were no adverse effects of anesthesia.

Enter three diagnosis codes and one procedure code.

PDX

DX2

DX3

PP1

AMBULATORY RECORD—PATIENT 4

PREOPERATIVE DIAGNOSIS: Reflex sympathetic dystrophy, left knee

POSTOPERATIVE DIAGNOSIS: Reflex sympathetic dystrophy, left knee

OPERATION: Left lumbar sympathetic block with C-arm

ANESTHESIA: Local

INDICATIONS:

This 43-year-old female has a 7-month history of left knee pain. She says that even a light touch appears to be exquisitely painful. She has had surgery to clear scar tissue.

PROCEDURE DESCRIPTION:

The patient was placed on the x-ray lucent gurney in the right lateral decubitus position. The back was prepped with Betadine, and the midline spinous processes were marked. A line was drawn 6 to 7 cm lateral to that midline on the left. L2 was identified using the C-arm and lateral projections, and lidocaine was infiltrated at the skin. The 22-gauge, 6-inch Chiba needle was advanced down to and off the body of L2, and loss of resistance was obtained with a glass syringe. Renografin-60 was injected and showed a good distribution. So 15 cc of bupivacaine 0.5% without epinephrine was injected, plus Depo-Medrol 40 mg. The needle was withdrawn.

Then lidocaine was infiltrated on the 6- to 7-cm line at L4. I advanced the 22-gauge, 6-inch needle off the body of L4, but the Renografin-60 distribution appeared not to be adequate. Another wheal was raised at the 13 level, and the needle was advanced down to and off the body of L3. A loss of resistance was obtained with a glass syringe, followed by Renografin-60. This time, the distribution was excellent, and bupivacaine 0.5% without epinephrine =15 cc was injected. She was left on her side for 25 minutes. After 10 minutes, she had a noticeably warmer left foot and ankle. The skin coloration of the left leg was normal.

Enter one diagnosis code and two procedure codes.

PDX

PP1

RR2

INPATIENT CASE—PATIENT 5

DATE OF ADMISSION: 1/5   **DATE OF DISCHARGE:** 1/7

DISCHARGE DIAGNOSIS:

1. Adenocarcinoma of the endometrium

2. Hemoperitoneum

3. Postoperative hemorrhage

4. Hypovolemic, hemorrhagic shock secondary to blood loss

COURSE IN HOSPITAL: The patient was taken to the operating room on 1/5 where a laparoscopically assisted vaginal hysterectomy was carried out.

At approximately 6:30 p.m. on the same day, I was called back into the hospital's recovery room because the patient was in shock with blood pressure of 80/60 with poor urine output and distended abdomen.

At this point it was decided to do an emergency diagnostic laparoscopy with preoperative diagnosis of postoperative hemorrhage. Bleeders were controlled with hemostatic sutures applied through the laparoscope.

The immediate postoperative course was essentially stormy with urine output maintained at 30 mL/h.

An ultrasound of the abdomen and pelvis was requested on the second postoperative day and this revealed normal renal shadow; no abnormal fluid accumulation in the pelvis or in the abdominal wall. The patient was then transferred to the regular floor on 1/6 after having maintained a satisfactory postoperative course from the second surgical procedure. The Jackson-Pratt drain was removed on 1/7 with closure of the abdominal incision with Steri-strips. The patient remained afebrile. She had been out of bed with good urine output and tolerating house diet. Her activities were increased gradually. Hemoglobin was again checked prior to discharge and was 12.1 g.

The patient was discharged to home on 1/7.

INSTRUCTIONS ON DISCHARGE: Regular diet. Follow up with appointment in my office in 3 days and with a colonoscopy for colon screening in light of family history of colon cancer.

HISTORY AND PHYSICAL EXAMINATION—PATIENT 5

ADMITTED: 1/5

REASON FOR ADMISSION: Vaginal bleeding

HISTORY OF PRESENT ILLNESS: This is a 62-year-old white female, gravida IV, para IV. She states that she has been in good health and has not had any gynecological complaints. During the past year she has had some left lower-quadrant pain and has noted post-coital bleeding. The bleeding has also occurred on and off for several months.

PAST MEDICAL HISTORY: Hypothyroidism due to thyroidectomy many years ago for benign tumor. No other serious illnesses, operations, or hospitalizations. The patient takes Synthroid 0.200 mcg.

ALLERGIES: No known drug or food allergies

CHRONIC MEDICATIONS: Synthroid 0.200 mcg

FAMILY HISTORY: Her mother died of colon cancer at age 53 years.

SOCIAL HISTORY: The patient is married with four children. She does not drink or smoke.

REVIEW OF SYSTEMS: HEENT essentially negative; wears glasses. Cardiorespiratory; no cough, dyspnea, cyanosis or chest pain. Gastrointestinal; no specific digestive or bowel complaints with the exception of the nonspecific left lower quadrant pain. The patient has no specific urinary complaints. The patient has a low hemoglobin level.

PHYSICAL EXAMINATION:

GENERAL APPEARANCE: Well-developed, well-nourished 62-year-old woman in no acute distress

HEENT: Essentially negative

LUNGS: Clear to P & A

HEART: Regular in force, rate, and rhythm. There are no audible murmurs.

ABDOMEN: No hernia or palpable masses. Abdomen is soft and flat. Peristalsis is normal. There are no areas of tenderness.

GENITALIA: Bimanual examination reveals the external genitalia to be normal. The uterus is of normal size. There are no palpable pelvic masses or tenderness.

RECTAL: Negative

IMPRESSION: Postmenopausal bleeding, possible endometrial carcinoma with blood loss anemia

PLAN: Vaginal hysterectomy

PROGRESS NOTES—PATIENT 5

DATE	NOTE

1/5 The patient is admitted for LAVH because of postmenopausal bleeding. She has also had left lower-quadrant pain. General condition is good.

Operative Note:

Preop: Possible adenocarcinoma of the endometrium

Postop: Same, pathology pending

Procedure: LAVH

Anesthesia: General

FINDINGS: Tubes and ovaries were within normal limits. Uterus is submitted for pathologic examination. Estimated blood loss is 300 cc. Called back to the RR for decrease in blood pressure and decreased urine output. The patient was found to have abdominal distention as well. The patient was given 3 units of blood and taken back to the operating room for evaluation of postoperative hemorrhage.

OPERATIVE NOTE:

1/5 Preop: Postop hemorrhage

Postop: Accidental laceration of epigastric artery, acute blood loss anemia

Procedure: Repair of bleeding vessel via laparoscope

Anesthesia: General

EBL: 1,500 to 2,000 mL of blood

The patient was admitted to the ICU following surgery where we will monitor her progress throughout the night.

1/6 Patient is doing well today. The BP is stable, urine output good—diuresing well, wound clean and dry, healing well. Will transfer her to the surgical floor.

1/7 The patient is stable, offers no complaints. Will discharge to home.

PHYSICIAN'S ORDERS—PATIENT 5

DATE	ORDER
1/5	Admit for LAVH
	Type and cross 4 units of blood, CBC
	Prepare for vaginal hysterectomy
	Synthroid 0.200 mcg daily
	NPO
	Demerol 75 mg
	Atropin 0.4 mg preop
	Postop, transfer patient to ICU
	D5NSS 125 cc/h
	Transfuse three units PRBC
	Demerol 75 mg IM q. 4 hours as need for pain
	Ancef 500 mg q. 6 hrs ×3 doses
	CBC q. 4 hrs, Strict I & O
1/6	Transfer to floor; please get patient OOB and provide liquids at bedside
	Continue I & O
	CBC this a.m. then tomorrow a.m.
	D/C IV after 6:00 p.m. if stable
1/7	Discharge to home

OPERATIVE REPORT—PATIENT 5

DATE: 1/5

PREOPERATIVE DIAGNOSIS: Possible adenocarcinoma of the endometrium

POSTOPERATIVE DIAGNOSIS: Pending pathology report

OPERATION: Laparoscopic assisted vaginal hysterectomy with pelvic cytology

ANESTHESIA: General

OPERATIVE PROCEDURE: With the patient under satisfactory general anesthesia in the semilithotomy position, she was prepped and draped in the usual fashion for a laparoscopic and vaginal procedure. Through an infraumbilical incision, a Veress needle was inserted to establish a pneumoperitoneum using a high-flow insufflator with CO_2 gas, maintaining 15 mm of pressure. It was then followed by insertion of a 10-mm trocar into the infraumbilical incision, followed by the laparoscope with laparoscopic examination having been done with findings described above.

After transillumination of the abdomen noting vessels, an incision was made in the skin and 12-mm trocars and sleeves were inserted into the right and left lower quadrant.

After having inserted the 12-mm sleeves, an endogauge was inserted into Channel A and levels of the right and left tubo-ovarian ligaments and broad ligaments were measured. An endo-GIA was then inserted into Channel A, followed by endo-GIA of Channel B, amputating the attachments of the tubes and ovaries and the broad ligaments. The remaining attachments of the board ligaments and the round ligaments were picked up with endo-GIA staplers on both sides.

A grasper was then inserted on Channel A, and the bladder reflection was picked up and elevated. It was then opened with endoshears, and using hydrodissection and ultrasonic scalpel, a bladder flap was created by sharp and blunt dissection with the scalpel. The dissection was carried down to the surface of the anterior lip of the cervix, which was noted to be smooth and free of adhesions. This was extended down past the cervicovaginal junction with identification of the tenaculum in the vagina. The grasper was then replaced on the right cornua and traction placed on the uterus, exposing the right cardinal ligaments, which was then placed on traction and using the scalpel probe, skeletonization of the uterine arteries with exposure of the arteries was done automatically.

The peritoneum was then dissected down past the uterosacral ligament insertion. After complete skeletonization of the uterine arteries was done, an endo TA-30 stapler was placed on the uterine arteries and the pedicle was cut off with the scalpel. There were no bleeding points noted.

The grasper was then removed and inserted into Channel B, and the left cornua of the uterus was picked up and placed on traction. The left cardinal ligaments and uterine arteries were then picked up and skeletonized, and complete exposure and dissection was done with visualization and identification of the arteries. The fragments of paravesical tissue were dissected off with the scalpel without traumatizing the bladder, which had previously been filled up with methylene blue and no spillage of the dye was noted during dissection of the uterus.

An endo TA-30 was then inserted in Channel A and linear staples were placed on the uterine arteries, on the left uterine artery and the cardinal ligament pedicles. The pedicle was then cut off with the scalpel. A second line of staples was then placed below the first line, taking care not to include the dome of the bladder without entering the vagina, and the pedicle cut off with the scalpel. There was a change in color of the uterus from pink to gray, indicating complete obliteration of blood supply.

OPERATIVE REPORT—PATIENT 5 (continued)

The staple lines on the infundibular pelvis ligaments were then inspected and this was found to be adequate. At this time the laparoscopic procedure was temporarily stopped and attention was then paid to the vaginal portion of the procedure, releasing the pneumoperitoneum that had been established for the laparoscopy. The cervix was exposed and picked up on the anterior a posterior lip with Lahey clamps, and a circumscribing incision was made on the cervicovaginal junction down to the level of the paravesical fascia and dissected off by sharp and blunt dissection with entry into the anterior cul-de-sac atraumatically, and the posterior cul-de-sac entered likewise.

The insertions of the base of the uterosacral ligaments and cardinal ligaments were then picked up with Heaney clamps, cut and suture ligated with #0 Vicryl, followed by a second line of Heaney clamps on the base of the remaining portion of the cardinal ligaments that was attached to the uterus, amputating and freeing up the uterus. The pedicles were tied off with #0 Vicryl materials and the uterus pulled and delivered out of the abdominal cavity through the vagina. Angle sutures were then placed on the vaginal cuff using #0 Vicryl material, and the intervening incision was closed with vertical mattress sutures using #0 Vicryl material.

After having closed the vagina and establishing adequate hemostasis, attention was once again placed on the laparoscopic portion. The pneumoperitoneum was once again established using high-flow insufflator and CO_2 gas at 10-mm pressure, and inspection and irrigation of the vascular pedicles and the vaginal cuff was done, which revealed them to be dry. The pelvis was irrigated with copious amounts of warm saline solution. The procedure was then terminated. The sleeve and gripper in Channel A was removed, and was found to be dry. The fascia was closed using an endo close needle with a #0 Vicryl suture in interrupted fashion using three stitches. The channel B 12-mm sheath and trocar were removed, which were dry.

At this time, termination of the procedure was done. The laparoscope was removed and the CO_2 released gradually. All instruments were removed and remaining stab wounds were closed in the fascia with #0 Vicryl sutures, and subcutaneously with #4-0 Monocryl. Sterile dressings were applied.

The patient was transferred to the recovery room in a reactive state with stable vital signs. Estimated blood loss was 300 mL of whole blood, no replacement given.

PATHOLOGY REPORT — PATIENT 5

DATE: 1/5

SPECIMEN: Uterus

CLINICAL DATA:

PREOPERATIVE DIAGNOSIS: Adenocarcinoma of endometrium

POSTOPERATIVE DIAGNOSIS: Same

GROSS DESCRIPTION: The specimen is labeled "Uterus." Submitted uterus with cervix attached. The specimen has previously been partially opened. It measures $9 \times 5 \times 3$ cm and weighs 58 g. The body of the uterus appears to be symmetrical. On section, the endocervix and ectocervix appear essentially normal. The endocervical canal likewise appears normal. The endometrial cavity is involved by a polypoid tumor mass chiefly in the right cornual area and measuring 3 cm in greatest diameter. The tumor appears to superficially penetrate the myometrium. The specimen will be further sectioned following fixation.

A and B are sections of cervix; C, D, E, F, G, and H are full-thickness section of tumor; section I is a full-thickness section from grossly uninvolved tissue.

MICROSCOPIC DESCRIPTION:

DIAGNOSIS: Adenocarcinoma, intermediate grade, of endometrium. Chronic cervicitis

COMMENT: The tumor penetrates approximately 0.4 cm into a total myometrial thickness of 1.5 cm.

OPERATIVE REPORT — PATIENT 5

DATE: 1/5

PREOPERATIVE DIAGNOSIS: Postoperative hemorrhage

POSTOPERATIVE DIAGNOSIS: Bleeding from right epigastric artery

OPERATION: Emergency diagnostic laparoscopy with repair of epigastric artery and blood transfusion

ANESTHESIA: General

OPERATIVE INDICATIONS: Estimated blood loss 1,500 to 2,000 mL of whole blood

OPERATIVE PROCEDURE: There was liquid and clotted blood in the abdominal cavity, approximately 1,500 to 2,000 mL, with blood coming from the puncture in the right lower quadrant, apparently from an accidental laceration of the right epigastric artery. The pedicles were inspected in the pelvis, and these were found to be dry.

With the patient under satisfactory general anesthesia, after having been transfused three units of packed RBCs, she was taken to the operating room and an emergency laparoscopic examination was carried out by opening the previous stab wounds with irrigation of the abdominal and pelvic cavity, evacuating approximately 1,500 to 2,000 mL of liquid and clotted blood.

Exposure of the pedicles of the infundibulopelvic ligament on both sides and the uterine arteries and the vaginal vault revealed them to be dry. There was no bleeding anywhere else in the pelvic cavity.

A puncture was found in the epigastric artery. Using an endoclosed needle through which a #0 Vicryl ligature was attached, the artery was repaired, stopping the bleeding point. This was verified by inspection with the laparoscope. After this was accomplished, the fascia was once again closed with endoclosed needle and #0 Vicryl suture on the right lower quadrant. The left lower quadrant was left open, and a Jackson-Pratt drain was inserted into the incision and placed in the pelvis for drainage.

The patient was then removed from the Trendelenburg position after ascertaining that vital signs were stable. The CO_2 was released gradually. All instruments were removed, and subcuticular closure of the stab wounds was done using #4-0 Monocryl sutures.

At the termination of surgery the patient's vital signs were stable. She, however, remained hypotensive with tachycardia with good urine output and was transfused an additional three units and transferred to the intensive care unit for postoperative care.

LABORATORY REPORTS — PATIENT 5

HEMATOLOGY

Specimen	Results				Normal Values
	1/5	1/5	1/5	1/7	
WBC	5.0	5.0	5.2	5.1	4.3–11.0
RBC	5.0	4.0 L	4.2 L	4.5	4.5–5.9
HGB	7.1 L	5.5 L	7.9 L	9.0 L	13.5–17.5
HCT	38 L	32 L	39 L	43	41–52
MCV	90	89	97	96	80–100
MCHC	44	46	48	50	31–57
PLT	160	165	170	300	150–400

LABORATORY REPORTS—PATIENT 5 *(continued)*

HEMATOLOGY—PATIENT 5

Specimen	Results				Normal Values
	1/5	1/5	1/5	1/7	
WBC	9.2	9.5	9.8	9.7	4.3–11.0
RBC	4.6	4.8	5.1	5.2	4.5–5.9
HGB	10.1 L	10.3 L	11.0 L	12.1 L	13.5–17.5
HCT	44	41	45	44	41–52
MCV	90	89	97	96	80–100
MCHC	44	46	48	50	31–57
PLT	160	165	170	300	150–400

Enter nine diagnosis codes and two procedure codes.

PDX

DX2

DX3

DX4

DX5

DX6

DX7

DX8

DX9

PP1

PR2

INPATIENT RECORD—PATIENT 6

DISCHARGE SUMMARY

DATE OF ADMISSION: 2/3   **DATE OF DISCHARGE:** 2/4

DISCHARGE DIAGNOSIS: Malignant ascites from metastatic adenocarcinoma of the colon

COURSE IN HOSPITAL: This 59-year-old white female patient was admitted for continuous infusion chemotherapy with 5-FU and Leucovoran. This was done under the care of Dr. ZXY. The patient tolerated her chemotherapy very well. She had no complications throughout her hospital course, and she was discharged to be followed further as an outpatient by her oncologist.

INSTRUCTIONS ON DISCHARGE: Follow up in the office.

HISTORY AND PHYSICAL EXAMINATION—PATIENT 6

ADMITTED: 2/3/20XX

REASON FOR ADMISSION: Chemotherapy

HISTORY OF PRESENT ILLNESS: The patient is a 59-year-old white female with carcinomatosis and malignant ascites from colon carcinoma. She is admitted for continuous chemotherapy. The patient has a sigmoid colostomy and has had multiple abdominal surgeries for carcinoma, the first one was an anterior and posterior repair in 1982. She had 6 weeks of radiation therapy completed two years ago and has been on weekly chemotherapy consisting of 5-FU and methotrexate recently. Because of increasing abdominal girth, she was admitted in June 1987, and diagnosed with malignant ascites and carcinomatosis. At that time, she had an extensive evaluation including an upper gastrointestinal series, barium enema, CT scan, and ultrasound of the abdomen. She was told she had adhesions causing a partial obstruction. No further surgery was pursued. For the past week, she has complained of frequent vomiting. Her weight has decreased another 6 pounds. She denies any abdominal pain. She has occasional diarrhea for which she takes Questran. She has had no blood in her colostomy drainage.

PAST MEDICAL HISTORY: No hypertension, myocardial infarction, diabetes, or peptic ulcer disease. Anterior and posterior repair in 1982, colectomy, cholecystectomy, appendectomy, hysterectomy with bilateral salpingo-oophorectomy for uterine fibroids in 1968.

ALLERGIES: None

CHRONIC MEDICATIONS: Pancrease three times a day; Questran as needed for diarrhea; Os-Cal 2 × per day, 250 mg

FAMILY HISTORY: Mother died at age 80. Father died of colon cancer at age 60.

SOCIAL HISTORY: She smoked a pack a day for 20 years. She denies any alcohol intake. She works in the shipping department.

REVIEW OF SYSTEMS: Unremarkable

PHYSICAL EXAMINATION: An alert, white female in no acute distress

HISTORY AND PHYSICAL EXAMINATION — PATIENT 6 (continued)

GENERAL APPEARANCE:

SKIN, HEAD, EYES, EARS, NOSE, THROAT: Pupils are equal, reactive to light and accommodation. Extraocular movements are intact. Fundi are benign. Tympanic membranes are normal.

MOUTH: No oral lesions are seen.

HEENT: Within normal limits

NECK: Carotids are plus 2 with no bruits. Thyroid is normal. There is no adenopathy at present.

LUNGS: Clear

HEART: Regular sinus rhythm. No murmur, rub, or gallop.

BREASTS: A small, approximately 3 mm, cystic lesion the medial aspect of her left breast at around eight o'clock. It is freely movable and nontender. There are no axillary nodes.

ABDOMEN: Distended. Sigmoid colostomy present. Right lower quadrant induration is present. There is no abdominal tenderness. There is no hepatosplenomegaly. Bowel sounds are normal.

PULSES: Femorals are plus 2 with no bruits. There are good pedal pulses bilaterally.

GENITALIA: Normal

RECTAL: Deferred

EXTREMITIES: No edema

NEUROLOGIC: Deep tendon reflexes are plus 2 throughout.

LABORATORY DATA: Pending

IMPRESSION:

Abdominal carcinomatosis retro-peritoneum and peritoneum from colon cancer

Small left breast cyst

PLAN: The patient will be admitted for continuous chemotherapy.

PROGRESS NOTES — PATIENT 6

DATE	NOTE
2/3	Patient tolerating chemo well. No complaints offered.
2/4	Patient well hydrated; nausea and vomiting under control. Will discharge.

PHYSICIAN'S ORDERS—PATIENT 6

DATE	ORDER
2/3	Chemotherapy protocol in D5W
	Compazine 5 mg now, then Q4H prn
2/4	Discontinue IV
	Discharge the patient.

Enter nine diagnosis codes and one procedure code.

PDX

DX2

DX3

DX4

DX5

DX6

DX7

DX8

DX9

PP1

INPATIENT RECORD—PATIENT 7

DISCHARGE SUMMARY

DATE OF ADMISSION: 9/8   **DATE OF DISCHARGE:** 9/10

DISCHARGE DIAGNOSIS:

1. Acute pyelonephritis

2. Septicemia, resistant to ampicillin and penicillin

ADMISSION HISTORY: This 21-year-old female was admitted to the hospital with discomfort in the right side. Other than this she has been healthy. On the day of admission she developed severe discomfort in the lower back. She was having fever and chills for which she took an aspirin and then she came to the emergency department.

COURSE IN HOSPITAL: The patient was treated with intravenous antibiotics in the form of gentamicin and cefoxitin. She continued to improve on this regimen and became afebrile after about three days of treatment. Her physical examination remained essentially unchanged; however, there was marked improvement in the patient's general condition. The patient also had an onset of herpes simplex infection on her upper lip, for which she was given Zovirax ointment.

INSTRUCTIONS ON DISCHARGE: The patient was discharged home on ciprofloxacin 500 mg p.o. b.i.d. × 12 days. A repeat blood culture done just prior to discharge showed no growth at the end of 7 days. She is to be followed up in my office in about a week after discharge to have a repeat urine culture done. The patient was also given a prescription for Zyban to assist smoking cessation.

HISTORY AND PHYSICAL EXAMINATION—PATIENT 7

ADMITTED: 9/8

REASON FOR ADMISSION: This was the first hospital admission for this 21-year-old white female, who experienced difficulty about 3 days prior to admission. This was in the form of discomfort in the right side of the lower back and also some dysuria. On the evening of admission, she started experiencing some fever and chills and took some aspirin. This did not help her and she came to the emergency department.

HISTORY OF PRESENT ILLNESS:

PAST MEDICAL HISTORY: Remarkable only for "walking pneumonia" treated with erythromycin 3 months ago. She also suffered contusion of her right kidney after a fall from a horse about 4 years prior to admission.

ALLERGIES: None known

CHRONIC MEDICATIONS: None

FAMILY HISTORY: Remarkable for multiple members of the family having seasonal allergies

SOCIAL HISTORY: The patient lives with two friends and is employed by a saddle shop. She drinks about one drink a week and smokes a pack of cigarettes a day.

REVIEW OF SYSTEMS: The patient relates that there has been no weight gain or loss and that she was well functioning until three days ago when she developed lower back pain, primarily on the right side. She also relates that she has had dysuria for this same time period.

HISTORY AND PHYSICAL EXAMINATION—PATIENT 7 (continued)

PHYSICAL EXAMINATION: On admission, significant for temperature of 103 degrees; pulse 120 beats per minute, regular; blood pressure 120/70; respirations 16

> **VITAL SIGNS:** P 120/min, regular; BP 120/70; Temp 103 degrees; R 16/min, regular
>
> **GENERAL:** The patient is a well-developed female of her stated age. She appears lethargic but responsive. The patient appears septic.
>
> **SKIN:** Warm to touch
>
> **HEENT:** Pupils equal, react briskly to light. Mucous membranes of the eyes, nose, mouth, and oropharynx are normal.
>
> **NECK:** Supple, trachea is central, the carotid pulses are symmetrical. There is no goiter.
>
> **LUNGS:** Clear to auscultation and percussion
>
> **BACK:** Positive pain to palpation and percussion right costovertebral angle
>
> **HEART:** Peripheral pulses are symmetrical. The cardiac apex is not displaced. The heart sounds are normal and there are no added sounds or murmurs.
>
> **ABDOMEN:** Soft, nontender, with no masses palpable. The bowel sounds are normal.
>
> **GENITALIA:** Normal female
>
> **RECTAL:** Deferred
>
> **EXTREMITIES:** Femoral pulses normal, no edema
>
> **NEUROLOGIC:** Grossly intact

LABORATORY DATA: WBC 15.9 with differential of 57 Segs; 33 Bands; 6 Lymphs; 4 Monos. Electrolytes were normal. BUN 11. Urine culture grew out *E. coli*, more than 100,000 colonies per mL. Blood culture was also positive for *E. coli*. This was sensitive to gentamicin and cefoxitin, as well as many other antibiotics. Urinalysis on admission revealed many WBCs and marked bacteriuria. Chest x-ray was unremarkable.

IMPRESSION: Admit for clinical features of acute pyelonephritis and septicemia.

PLAN: Hydrate and start IV antibiotics.

PROGRESS NOTES—PATIENT 7

DATE	NOTE
9/8	Patient admitted for evaluation of flank pain and fever. She also has a lesion on her lip. This appears to be herpes simplex. Will treat infection process with antibiotics following obtaining cultures. The patient's renal function will be monitored.
9/10	The patient's fever decreasing. Patient comfortable and tolerating antibiotics. Will continue IVs. The importance of stopping cigarette use was discussed with the patient. She is willing to quit and she will be given a prescription for Zyban at discharge.
9/11	Patient is afebrile today. Will discharge when able to obtain transportation.

PHYSICIAN'S ORDERS—PATIENT 7

DATE	ORDER
9/8	Admit to floor for evaluation of febrile illness
	Urinalysis
	CBC and SMA 16
	Urine culture and sensitivity
	Blood cultures ×2
	Chest x-ray
	Pyelogram
	D5W 125 cc/h ×3
	Strict input and output
	Zovirax ointment prn to lip
	Gentamicin 80 mg IV q. 8 H ×3d
	Cefoxitin 1 g IV q. 8 H ×3 days
9/9	D5W 100 cc/ph
9/10	Discharge patient when transportation is arranged
	Ciprofloxacin 500 mg p.o. b.i.d. ×12 days
	Zyban 150 mg p.o. daily ×3 days then b.i.d.
	Follow up in the office in 1 week.

LABORATORY REPORTS—PATIENT 7

HEMATOLOGY

DATE: 9/8

Specimen	Results	Normal Values
WBC	15.9 H	4.3–11.0
RBC	5.5	4.5–5.9
HGB	14.0	13.5–17.5
HCT	45	41–52
MCV	90	80–100
MCHC	41	31–57
PLT	251	150–450

LABORATORY REPORTS — PATIENT 7 (continued)

CHEMISTRY—PATIENT 7

DATE: 9/8

Specimen	Results	Normal Values
GLUC	100	70–110
BUN	11	8–25
CREAT	1.0	0.5–1.5
NA	143	136–146
K	4.0	3.5–5.5
CL	98	95–110
CO_2	30	24–32
CA	9.0	8.4–10.5
PHOS	3.0	2.5–4.4
MG	2.0	1.6–3.0
T BILI	1.0	0.2–1.2
D BILI	0.3	0.0–0.5
PROTEIN	7.0	6.0–8.0
ALBUMIN	5.2	5.0–5.5
AST	25	0–40
ALT	40	30–65
GGT	60	15–85
LD		100–190
ALK PHOS		50–136
URIC ACID		2.2–7.7
CHOL		0–200
TRIG		10–160

URINALYSIS—PATIENT 7

DATE: 9/8

Test	Result	Ref Range
SP GRAVITY	1.03	1.005–1.035
PH	6	5–7
PROT	NEG	NEG
GLUC	NEG	NEG
KETONES	NEG	NEG
BILI	NEG	NEG
BLOOD	NEG	NEG
LEU EST	POS	NEG
NITRATES	POS	NEG
RED SUBS	NEG	NEG

MICROBIOLOGY—PATIENT 7

DATE	**TEST TYPE:** Culture and Sensitivity
9/8	SOURCE: Urine
	SITE:
	GRAM STAIN RESULTS
	CULTURE RESULTS: *E. coli*, 100,000/ml
	SUSCEPTIBILITY:

9/10		
AMPICILLIN	R
CEFAZOLIN	S
CEFOTAXIME	S
CEFTRIAXONE	S
CEFUROXIME	S
CEPHALOTHIN	S
CIPROFLOXACIN	S
ERYTHROMYCIN	S
GENTAMICIN	S
OXACILLIN	S
PENICILLIN	R
PIPERACILLIN	
TETRACYCLINE	
TOBRAMYCIN	
TRIMETH/SULF	
VANCOMYCIN	

S = SUSCEPTIBLE

R = RESISTANT

I = INTERMEDIATE

M = MODERATELY SUSCEP

LABORATORY RESULTS—PATIENT 7

DATE: 9/11

URINE CULTURE: No growth for 24 hours

MICROBIOLOGY — PATIENT 7

DATE	TEST TYPE:	
9/8	Culture and Sensitivity #1	
	SOURCE: Blood	
	SITE:	
	GRAM STAIN RESULTS	
	CULTURE RESULTS: *E. coli*	
	SUSCEPTIBILITY:	
9/10	AMPICILLIN	R
	CEFAZOLIN	S
	CEFOTAXIME	S
	CEFTRIAXONE	S
	CEFUROXIME	S
	CEPHALOTHIN	S
	CIPROFLOXACIN	S
	ERYTHROMYCIN	S
	GENTAMICIN	S
	OXACILLIN	S
	PENICILLIN	R
	PIPERACILLIN	
	TETRACYCLINE	
	TOBRAMYCIN	
	TRIMETH/SULF	
	VANCOMYCIN	

S = SUSCEPTIBLE

R = RESISTANT

I = INTERMEDIATE

M = MODERATELY SUSCEP

MICROBIOLOGY — PATIENT 7

DATE	TEST TYPE:
9/8	Culture and Sensitivity #2
	SOURCE: Blood
	SITE:
	GRAM STAIN RESULTS
	CULTURE RESULTS: *E. coli*
	SUSCEPTIBILITY:

9/10		
	AMPICILLIN	R
	CEFAZOLIN	S
	CEFOTAXIME	S
	CEFTRIAXONE	S
	CEFUROXIME	S
	CEPHALOTHIN	S
	CIPROFLOXACIN	S
	ERYTHROMYCIN	S
	GENTAMICIN	S
	OXACILLIN	S
	PENICILLIN	R
	PIPERACILLIN	
	TETRACYCLINE	
	TOBRAMYCIN	
	TRIMETH/SULF	
	VANCOMYCIN	

S = SUSCEPTIBLE

R = RESISTANT

I = INTERMEDIATE

M = MODERATELY SUSCEP

RADIOLOGY REPORT — PATIENT 7

DATE: 9/8

CHEST X-RAY: The examination is of a recumbent AP view. Heart size is normal. The aorta is normal and lung fields are free of infiltration. There is no free air and the trachea is midline.

DIAGNOSIS: Normal chest x-ray

RADIOLOGY REPORT — PATIENT 7

DATE: 9/8

PYELOGRAM: The urinary architecture is normal with no hydronephrosis.

DIAGNOSIS: Normal pyelogram

Enter five diagnosis codes.

PDX

DX2

DX3

DX4

DX5

PRACTICE EXAM 1

A blank answer sheet for these multiple choice questions can be found on page 98.

Domain I *Health Information Documentation*

1. A 7-year-old patient was admitted to the emergency department for treatment of shortness of breath. The patient is given epinephrine and nebulizer treatments. The shortness of breath and wheezing are unabated following treatment. What diagnosis should be suspected?

   a. Acute bronchitis

   b. Acute bronchitis with chronic obstructive pulmonary disease

   c. Asthma with status asthmaticus

   d. Chronic obstructive asthma

2. A patient is admitted with a high temperature, lethargy, hypotension, tachycardia, oliguria, and elevated WBC. The patient also has more than 100,000 organisms of *Escherichia coli* per cc of urine. The attending physician documents "urosepsis." What is the next step for the coder?

   a. Code sepsis as the principal with a secondary diagnosis of urinary tract infection due to *E. coli*.

   b. Code urinary tract infection with sepsis as a secondary diagnosis.

   c. Query the physician to determine if the patient is being treated for sepsis, highlighting the clinical signs and symptoms.

   d. Ask the physician whether the patient had septic shock so that this may be used as the principal diagnosis.

3. During a coronary artery bypass surgery, the patient underwent saphenous bypass grafts; from the aorta to the left anterior descending branch of the left main coronary artery, and the left posterior descending of the left main coronary artery. The patient also underwent a repositioning of the mammary artery to the right coronary artery. Choose the best description for this procedure.

   a. Three aortocoronary grafts

   b. Two aortocoronary grafts and one mammary-coronary graft

   c. Two aortocoronary grafts and two saphenous bypass graft

   d. Three aortocoronary grafts and one mammary-coronary graft

4. According to CPT, an endoscopy that is undertaken to the level of the midtransverse colon would be coded as a:

   a. Proctosigmoidoscopy

   b. Sigmoidoscopy

   c. Colonoscopy

   d. Proctoscopy

5. Infusion of Herceptin which is a monoclonal antibody used for treatment of breast cancer in patients carrying a certain mutation of the HER2 gene is classified as:

   a. Chemotherapy

   b. Radiotherapy

   c. Genotherapy

   d. Immunotherapy

6. A patient has findings suggestive of chronic obstructive pulmonary disease (COPD) on chest x-ray. The attending physician mentions the x-ray finding in one progress note but no medication, treatment, or further evaluation is provided. The coder should:

   a. Query the attending physician regarding the x-ray finding

   b. Code the condition because the documentation reflects it

   c. Question the radiologist regarding whether to code this condition

   d. Use a code from abnormal findings to reflect the condition

7. If a patient undergoes an inpatient procedure and the final summary diagnosis is different from the diagnosis on the pathology report, the coder should:

   a. Code only from the discharge diagnoses

   b. Code the diagnosis reflected on the pathology report

   c. Code the most severe symptom

   d. Query the attending physician as to the final diagnosis

8. A 56-year-old woman is admitted to an acute-care facility from a skilled nursing facility. The patient has multiple sclerosis and hypertension. During the course of hospitalization a decubitus ulcer is found and debrided at the bedside by a physician. There is no typed operative report and no pathology report. The coder should:

   a. Use an excisional debridement code as these charts are rarely reviewed to verify the excisional debridement

   b. Code with a nonexcisional debridement procedure code

   c. Query the healthcare provider who performed the procedure to determine if the debridement was excisional

   d. Eliminate the procedure code all together

9. A 23-year-old female is admitted for shock following treatment of a miscarriage. The pathology report from the previous admission reveals that the patient had no decidua or products of conception in the tissue removed. This encounter would be coded as:

   a. 634, Spontaneous abortion

   b. 639, Complication following abortion and ectopic and molar pregnancies

   c. 785.50, Shock NOS

   d. 998.0, Postoperative shock

10. Most hospitals require a medical record is completed within:

   a. 5 days

   b. 10 days

   c. 7 days

   d. 30 days

11. To correct an entry in the record, the provider should:

   a. Draw a single line through the error, add a note explaining the error, initial and date, add the correct information in chronological order

   b. Draw a double line through the error, initial and date, add the reason for the correction

   c. Draw a single line through the error, and add the correct information in chronological order

   d. Draw several lines through the error, obliterate the documentation as much as possible, initial and date, add the correct information in chronological order

12. After a patient is discharged from the hospital, the medical record must be reviewed for:

   a. Inclusion of all incident reports

   b. Certain basic reports (for example history and physical, discharge summary, etc.)

   c. Voided prescription pads

   d. Personal case notes from all mental health providers

Domain II *Diagnosis & Procedure Coding*

13. A patient is admitted for chest pain. The patient was stabilized and discharged. In a subsequent admission, the patient was admitted as an outpatient for a left heart catheterization, coronary arteriography using two catheters and left ventricular angiography. The patient was found to have arteriosclerotic heart disease. The patient has no history of cardiac surgery. The appropriate sequencing of ICD-9 and CPT codes for the outpatient catheterization would be:

411.1	Intermediate coronary syndrome (unstable angina)
413.9	Other and unspecified angina pectoris
414.00	Coronary atherosclerosis of unspecified type of vessel, native or graft
414.01	Coronary atherosclerosis of native coronary artery
786.50	Chest pain, unspecified
93452	Left heart catheterization including intraprocedural injection(s) for left ventriculography, imaging supervision and interpretation, when performed
93453	Combined right and left heart catheterization including intraprocedural injection(s) for left ventriculography, imaging supervision and interpretation, when performed
93454	Catheter placement in coronary artery(s) for coronary angiography, including intraprocedural injection(s) for coronary angiography, imaging supervision and interpretation;
93458	with left heart catheterization including intraprocedural injection(s) for left ventriculography, when performed

   a. 786.50, 93452

   b. 411.1, 93454

   c. 414.01, 413.9, 93453

   d. 414.01, 93458

14. A 65-year-old patient is admitted with pain and loosening of a previous total hip arthroplasty. The acetabular component has loosened and become painful. The patient was admitted for revision of the hip replacement. The acetabular component uses a metal-on-metal bearing surface. What is the appropriate code(s) for the admission?

996.41	Mechanical loosening of prosthetic joint
996.66	Infection and inflammatory reaction due to internal joint prosthesis
V43.64	Organ or tissue replaced by other means, hip
00.71	Revision of hip replacement, acetabular component
00.74	Hip-bearing surface, metal on polyethylene
00.75	Hip-bearing surface, metal on metal
00.76	Hip-bearing surface, ceramic on ceramic

a. 996.41, V43.64, 00.71, 00.75

b. 996.66, 00.75

c. 996.41, V43.64, 00.71

d. 996.66, V43.64, 00.71, 00.75

15. A maternity patient is admitted in labor at 43 weeks. She has a normal delivery with vacuum extraction to facilitate the baby's delivery. Which of the following would be the principal diagnosis?

650	Normal delivery
645.11	Post-term pregnancy, delivered, with or without mention of antepartum condition
645.21	Prolonged pregnancy, delivered, with or without mention of antepartum condition
669.51	Forceps or vacuum extractor delivery without mention of indication, delivered, with or without mention of antepartum condition

a. 645.11

b. 645.21

c. 650

d. 669.51

16. With regard to the implementation of ICD-10-CM, all of the following are correct *except*:

a. ICD-10-CM was developed by NCHS

b. ICD-10-CM and ICD-10-PCS will be fully implemented beginning October 1, 2012

c. ICD-10 is already being used in the United States for death certificate coding

d. The process of adoption of ICD-10-CM is specified in HIPAA

17. A 75-year-old female was admitted for acute myocardial infarction and underwent a diagnostic cardiac catheterization. Following the catheterization, the patient developed a pseudoaneurysm documented as due to the catheterization in the common femoral artery. The pseudoaneurysm would be coded as:

    a. 997.2, Peripheral vascular complication
       442.3, Other aneurysm of artery of lower extremity

    b. 998.2, Accidental puncture or laceration during a procedure
       442.3, Other aneurysm of artery of lower extremity

    c. 442.3, Other aneurysm of artery of lower extremity

    d. 998.2, Accidental puncture or laceration during a procedure

18. A patient was admitted to the emergency department with chest pain, and was diagnosed with aborted myocardial infarction with acute myocardial ischemia. There was no prior cardiac surgery. The cardiac enzymes were normal. The appropriate coding of the diagnosis for this case is:

    a. 410.91, Acute myocardial infarction, unspecified site

    b. 414.01, Coronary atherosclerosis of native coronary artery

    c. 411.89, Other acute and subacute forms of ischemic heart disease

    d. 411.81, Acute coronary occlusion without myocardial infarction

19. A patient has nausea and vomiting with abdominal pain due to acute cholecystitis. The physician documents the following on the discharge summary: acute cholecystitis, nausea, vomiting, and abdominal pain. The diagnosis(es) that would be coded is(are):

    a. Acute cholecystitis, nausea, vomiting, and abdominal pain

    b. Acute cholecystitis, nausea, vomiting

    c. Acute cholecystitis, nausea

    d. Acute cholecystitis

20. A patient is admitted because of congestive heart failure (CHF). During the treatment of the CHF the patient was also found to have elevated liver function tests. The physician worked up the elevated liver function tests but was not able to determine a diagnosis with regard to the abnormal liver tests. The coder should identify the following diagnosis(es) when coding the record:

    a. Congestive heart failure with liver disease

    b. Abnormal liver function tests

    c. Congestive heart failure and a code from the findings abnormal section

    d. Congestive heart failure

21. A patient is admitted with hypotension due to dobutamine taken, administered, and prescribed correctly. How should this be coded?

    a. 458.0, Orthostatic hypotension
       E941.2, Adverse effects of dobutamine

    b. 458.29, Other iatrogenic hypotension
       E941.2, Adverse effects of dobutamine

    c. 458.8, Other specified hypotension
       E941.2, Adverse effects of dobutamine

    d. 458.1, Chronic hypotension
       E941.2, Adverse effects of dobutamine

22. A patient is readmitted two weeks after a laminectomy for spinal stenosis with a headache due to a defect in the dura accidently caused during surgery. The patient is taken to the operating room for repair of the dura. The code(s) assigned for this admission would be:

    a. 724.02, Spinal stenosis, lumbar region, without neurogenic claudication

    b. 349.31, Accidental puncture or laceration of dura during a procedure
       349.0, Spinal fluid loss headache

    c. 952.2, Laceration of dura

    d. 724.02, Spinal stenosis, lumbar region, without neurogenic claudication
       952.2, Laceration of dura

23. A patient is admitted to the hospital with shortness of breath and congestive heart failure and subsequently develops respiratory failure. The patient undergoes intubation with ventilator management. The correct coding and sequencing of the diagnoses in this case would be:

    a. Congestive heart failure, respiratory failure, ventilator management, intubation

    b. Respiratory failure, intubation, ventilator management

    c. Respiratory failure, congestive heart failure, intubation, ventilator management

    d. Shortness of breath, congestive heart failure, respiratory failure, ventilator management, intubation

24. If a patient is admitted with pneumococcal pneumonia and pneumococcal sepsis, the coder should:

    a. Assign a code for only the sepsis and pneumonia

    b. Assign a code for the sepsis, pneumonia, and SIRS

    c. Assign only a code for pneumococcal pneumonia

    d. Review the chart to determine if septic shock could be used first

25. A patient was admitted with end stage renal disease (ESRD) following kidney transplant. The patient also had angina and chronic obstructive pulmonary disease. The diagnoses would be coded and sequenced as:

    a. Kidney failure; status post kidney transplant; chronic obstructive pulmonary disease; angina

    b. End-stage renal disease; status post kidney transplant; chronic obstructive pulmonary disease; angina

    c. Chronic kidney disease, stage V; status post kidney transplant; chronic obstructive pulmonary disease; angina

    d. Acute kidney failure; status post kidney transplant; chronic obstructive pulmonary disease; angina

26. A patient is admitted to the hospital because of a fracture of the right hip and is scheduled for an open reduction with internal fixation of a hip fracture. The patient developed a cardiac arrhythmia which results in an inability to do the planned surgery. Assign a code for the principal diagnosis.

    a. Status post fracture

    b. Cardiac arrhythmia

    c. Fracture of the right

    d. Admission for possible fracture

27. Which of the following is *not* part of a facility coding compliance plan?

    a. Regular internal audits

    b. Audits performed by objective external reviewers

    c. Coding audits performed by payers

    d. Sharing and discussing results with coding staff

28. In CPT, unlisted codes are reported only if:

    a. There is not a current CPT category I code available

    b. There is not a current CPT category III code available

    c. There is not a current CPT category II code available

    d. There is not a current CPT category I or III code available

29. A virtual screening colonoscopy would be coded as:

45378	Colonoscopy, flexible, proximal to splenic flexure; diagnostic, with or without collection of specimen(s) by brushing or washing, with or without colon decompression (separate procedure)
45391	Colonoscopy, flexible, proximal to splenic flexure; with endoscopic ultrasound examination
74263	Computed tomographic (CT) colonography, screening including image postprocessing.
76376	3D rendering with interpretation and reporting of computed tomography, magnetic resonance imaging, ultrasound, or other tomographic modality with image post-processing under concurrent supervision; not requiring image postprocessing on an independent workstation

    a. 74263

    b. 45391

    c. 45378

    d. 76376

30. A patient underwent an excision of a malignant lesion of the chest that measured 1.0 cm and there was a 0.2 cm margin on both sides. Based on the 2011 CPT codes, which code would be used for the procedure?

    a. 11401, Excision benign lesion of trunk … excised diameter 0.6 cm to 1.0 cm

    b. 11601, Excision malignant lesion of trunk … excised diameter 0.6 cm to 1.0 cm

    c. 11602, Excision malignant lesion of trunk … excised diameter 1.1 cm to 2.0 cm

    d. 11402, Excision benign lesion of trunk … excised diameter 1.1 cm to 2.0 cm

31. A patient was diagnosed with L4-5 lumbar neuropathy and discogenic pain. The patient underwent an intradiscal electrothermal annuloplasty (IDET) in the radiology suite. What ICD-9-CM code should be used?

    a. 80.50, Excision, destruction and other repair of intervertebral disc, unspecified

    b. 04.2, Destruction of cranial and peripheral nerves

    c. 80.59, Other destruction of intervertebral disc

    d. 05.23, Lumbar sympathectomy

32. A laparoscopic tubal ligation with Falope ring is completed. What is the correct CPT code assignment?

49321	Laparoscopy, surgical; with biopsy (single or multiple)
58662	Laparoscopy, surgical; with fulguration or excision of lesions of the ovary, pelvic viscera, or peritoneal surface by any method
58670	Laparoscopy, surgical; with fulguration of oviducts (with or without transection)
58671	Laparoscopy, surgical; with occlusion of oviducts by device (eg, band, clip, or Falope ring)

a. 49321, 58662

b. 58670

c. 58671

d. 49321

33. Carcinoma of multiple overlapping sites of the bladder. Diagnostic cystoscopy and transurethral fulguration of bladder lesions (1.9 cm, 6.0 cm) are undertaken. The appropriate CPT code(s) would be:

52000	Cystourethroscopy (separate procedure)
52224	Cystourethroscopy, with fulguration (including cryosurgery or laser surgery) or treatment of minor (less than 0.5 cm) lesion(s) with or without biopsy
52234	Cystourethroscopy, with fulguration (including cryosurgery or laser surgery) and/or resection of small bladder tumor(s) (0.5 cm to 2.0 cm)
52235	Cystourethroscopy, with fulguration (including cryosurgery or laser surgery) and/or resection of medium bladder tumor(s) (2.0 cm to 5.0 cm)
52240	Cystourethroscopy, with fulguration (including cryosurgery or laser surgery) and/or resection of large bladder tumor(s)

a. 52234, 52240

b. 52235

c. 52240

d. 52000, 52234

34. A patient presents to a facility for upper endoscopy implant of material into the muscle of the lower esophageal sphincter. The correct coding and sequencing of this patient's record is:

43235	Upper gastrointestinal endoscopy including esophagus, stomach, and either the duodenum and/or jejunum as appropriate; diagnostic, with or without collection of specimen(s) by brushing or washing (separate procedure)
43257	with delivery of thermal energy to the muscle of lower esophageal sphincter and/or gastric cardia, for treatment of gastroesophageal reflux disease
43258	with ablation of tumor(s) polyp(s), or other lesion(s) not amenable to removal by hot biopsy forceps, bipolar cautery or snare technique
43236	with directed submucosal injection(s), any substance
−59	Distinct procedure service

a. 43257

b. 43235, 43236

c. 43236

d. 43258, 43236−59

35. A patient undergoes a colposcopy with endometrial biopsy. Which of the following is correct?

    a. The colposcopy and endometrial biopsy are represented by a combination code.

    b. Two codes would be used with modifier –59 appended.

    c. Two codes would be used in accordance with 2013 CPT code revisions.

    d. Only one code is used and it does not state that it includes endometrial biopsy specifically.

36. A patient presents to the outpatient surgical area for a cystoscopy with multiple biopsies of the bladder. The patient's presenting symptom is hematuria. What is the correct code assignment for this procedure?

52000	Cystourethroscopy (separate procedure)
52204	Cystourethroscopy with biopsy(s)
–22	Increased procedural services

    a. 52000

    b. 52000–22

    c. 52204

    d. 52204–22

37. If a patient has an excision of a malignant lesion of the skin, the CPT code is determined by the body area from which the excision occurs and the:

    a. Length of the lesion as described in the pathology report

    b. Dimension of the specimen submitted as described in the pathology report

    c. Width times the length of the lesion as described in the operative report

    d. Diameter of the lesion as well as the margins excised as described in the operative report

38. When coding "arthrocentesis," the code assignment is determined by:

    a. Contrast used

    b. Size of the joint

    c. Approach

    d. Description of the closure

Domain III *Regulatory Guidelines and Reporting Requirements for Acute-Care (Inpatient) Service*

39. Documentation in the record reveals that a patient is admitted with an acute exacerbation of COPD (MS-DRG 192). A higher-paying DRG may be appropriate if documentation is present in the record at the time the decision was made to admit the patient that confirms a diagnosis associated with which of the following:

    a. Angina was treated with nitroglycerin prn for chest pain

    b. Atrial fibrillation and underwent a cardioversion while hospitalized

    c. Blood gases of pO_2 of 58, pCO_2 of 55, pH of 7.32 upon admission and treated with intubation and mechanical ventilation for more than 96 hours

    d. Anemia and was given a blood transfusion

40. A female patient is diagnosed with congestive heart failure. Which of the following will increase the MS-DRG weight if present on admission?

    a. Atrial fibrillation

    b. Stage III pressure ulcer

    c. Blood loss anemia

    d. Coronary artery disease

41. If the principal diagnosis is an initial episode of an anterior wall myocardial infarction, which procedure will result in the highest DRG?

    a. Mechanical ventilator

    b. Insertion central venous catheter

    c. Right heart cardiac catheterization

    d. Transbronchial lung biopsy

42. Patient admitted with hemorrhage due to placenta previa with twin pregnancy. This patient had two prior (cesarean section) deliveries. Emergent C-section delivery was performed due to the hemorrhage. The appropriate principal diagnosis would be:

    a. Prior cesarean sections

    b. Placenta previa without hemorrhage

    c. Twin gestation

    d. Placenta previa with hemorrhage

43. A patient is admitted with spotting and fever. She is found to have been treated for a miscarriage (spontaneous abortion), which was resolved two weeks prior to this admission. She is treated with aspiration dilation and curettage and products of conception are found. She is found to be septic. Which of the following should be the principal diagnosis?

    a. Complications following abortion and ectopic or other pregnancy

    b. Complications of spontaneous abortion with sepsis

    c. Sepsis

    d. Incomplete spontaneous abortion with sepsis

44. A patient is admitted with an acute inferior myocardial infarction and discharged alive. Which condition would increase the MS-DRG weight?

    a. Respiratory failure

    b. Atrial fibrillation

    c. Hypertension

    d. History of myocardial infarction

45. A 70-year-old patient was admitted with pneumonia. The history and physical documented that the patient has a history of diabetes, hypertension, and migraine headache about 10 years ago without recurrence. The patient was administered IV antibiotics, metformin, and Altace during the hospitalization. Which conditions would be reported at the time of discharge?

    a. Pneumonia, diabetes, hypertension, and migraine headaches

    b. Pneumonia, diabetes, hypertension, and history of migraine headaches

    c. Pneumonia, diabetes, and hypertension

    d. Pneumonia

46. A diabetic patient was admitted for a treatment of a pressure ulcer. The patient also has a history of diabetic neuropathy and retinopathy. The patient is blind and additional nursing care and extended time with the patient was required. Which conditions should be coded at discharge?

    a. Pressure ulcer, history of neurologic condition, history of retinal condition, diabetes

    b. Pressure ulcer, diabetic neuropathy and diabetic retinopathy, and blindness

    c. Pressure ulcer, diabetic neuropathy

    d. Pressure ulcer, diabetic retinopathy, and blindness

47. During an admission for CHF a chest x-ray was done to evaluate for the presence of congestive heart failure (CHF). An asymptomatic hernia was also found for which *no* treatment or evaluation was done. What is the primary reason that the hernia should not be coded?

    a. The patient's primary condition of interest is the CHF

    b. The hernia is an incidental finding

    c. The patient is asymptomatic

    d. The condition does not impact the reimbursement.

48. When an inpatient has had multiple tests to evaluate an abnormal finding but no definitive diagnosis has been documented the coder should:

    a. Assign a code for the abnormal finding

    b. Assign codes for all of the abnormal results of the tests

    c. Assign a diagnosis code based on the coder's judgment

    d. Query the physician regarding whether a diagnosis should be assigned or not

Domain IV   *Regulatory Guidelines and Reporting Requirements for Outpatient Services*

Use the information in this table to answer questions 49 through 51.

Billing Number	Status Indicator	CPT/HCPCS	APC*
989323	V	99285–25	00616
989323	T	25500	00129
989323	X	72050	00261
989323	S	72128	08005
989323	N	70450	19937

*This is not the actual reimbursement for the designated APC.

49. From the information provided, how many APCs would impact this patient's total reimbursement?

    a. 1

    b. 5

    c. 4

    d. Unable to determine

50. What percentage will the facility be paid for procedure code 25500?

    a. 50%

    b. 75%

    c. 0%

    d. 100%

51. If another status T procedure were performed, how much would the facility receive for the second status T procedure?

    a. 50%

    b. 75%

    c. 0%

    d. 100%

52. When a Medicare patient receives an injection of IM penicillin G benzathine, 100,000 units only, what is the appropriate code assignment?

96372	Therapeutic, prophylactic or diagnostic injection (specify substance or drug); subcutaneous or intramuscular
96374	Therapeutic, prophylactic or diagnostic injection (specify substance or drug); intravenous push, single or initial substance/drug
J0558	Injection, penicillin G benzathine, and penicillin G procaine 100,000 units
J0561	Injection, penicillin G benzathine, 100,000 units

    a. 96372

    b. J0558

    c. 96374

    d. 96372, J0561

53. Determining medical necessity for outpatient services includes all the following *except*:

    a. Local coverage determinations (LCDs)

    b. National coverage determinations (NCDs)

    c. Diagnoses linked to procedures by claims-processing software tests ensuring that the procedure is cross-referenced, or linked, correctly to an acceptable diagnosis code for that service

    d. Requiring new HCPCS codes be developed to replace codes in the CPT code book

54. According to the UHDDS, section III, the definition of *other diagnoses* is all conditions that:

    a. Coexist at the time of admission, that develop subsequently, or that affect the treatment received and/or the length of stay

    b. Receive evaluation and is documented by the physician

    c. Receive clinical evaluation, therapeutic treatment, further evaluation, extend the length of stay, increase nursing monitoring/care

    d. Are considered to be essential by the physicians involved and are reflected in the record

55. If a patient has undergone an outpatient echocardiogram and the cardiologist concludes in the report that the patient has mitral regurgitation the coder should:

    a. Assign a diagnostic code for mitral regurgitation

    b. Query the physician about the diagnosis

    c. Code an abnormal finding of the echocardiogram

    d. No code can be assigned

56. During an ambulatory surgery visit for excision of a malignant melanoma of the right forearm, the attending surgeon listed history of benign breast cyst, history of hypertension currently on Tenormin, and a current hammer toe. Which conditions are to be coded?

    a. Malignant melanoma of forearm, hypertension

    b. Malignant melanoma of the right forearm, benign breast cyst, hypertension and hammer toe

    c. Malignant melanoma of the right forearm, benign breast cyst, and hypertension

    d. Malignant melanoma of the right forearm, benign breast cyst

57. A chest x-ray done to evaluate a chronic cough revealed a asymptomatic compression fracture of a lumbar vertebrae. No further evaluation was undertaken. The coder should:

    a. Not assign a code for an acute condition but assign a code for chronic compression fracture

    b. Assign a code for pathologic lumbar compression fracture

    c. Assign a code for acute traumatic vertebral fracture

    d. Not assign a code for this condition

58. During an outpatient visit the attending physician did not define a problem at the conclusion of an emergency department (ED) visit. The coder should:

    a. Assign a code from the list of conditions in the history that occurred in the past

    b. Assign a code for the reason for the last visit to the ED

    c. Assign codes for abnormal laboratory findings

    d. Assign a code for the chief complaint as the reason for the visit

Domain V *Data Quality and Management*

59. The outpatient code editor (OCE) has all of the following types of edits *except*:

    a. Claim accuracy

    b. Discharge date discrepancy

    c. Assigning APCs to the claim

    d. Age and sex edits

Refer to the following data when answering questions 60 and 61. (Note: The DRG weights are not actual weights for fiscal year 2013.)

MS-DRG	MS-DRG Weight	Number of Patients
MS-DRG 193, Simple pneumonia and pleurisy age >17 w/ CC	3.0	10
MS-DRG 195, Simple pneumonia without MCC or CC	2.0	10
MS-DRG 192, Chronic obstructive pulmonary disease w/o CC	1.0	10

60. The case-mix index for the information provided above is:

    a. 0.679

    b. 0.89

    c. 2.0

    d. 0.75

61. The information provided shows that:

    a. The payment is higher for patients with pneumonia with CCs than without

    b. There are more patients with pneumonia without MCCs than with MCCs

    c. There is a large pediatric population at this hospital with pneumonia

    d. There is inaccurate coding of pneumonia at this institution

62. A nurse inadvertently recorded an incorrect vital sign in a patient electronic health record. The next day, a correction was made in the electronic health record. This resulted in the corrected vital sign being recorded at the time the correction was made due to the software. What would be the result of this correction?

    a. The vital signs would be listed in the correct sequence.

    b. When a correction is made in an electronic health record, the incorrect data is deleted.

    c. The quality of patient care would not be affected.

    d. There was a distorted trend line of vital signs data.

63. According to the UHDDS, in order to assign a code for another diagnosis, documentation must be present that:

a. The condition is recorded in the patient record by a dietary clerk

b. The condition is present in the admission department data

c. The condition was clinically evaluated or therapeutically treated, extended the length of hospital stay or increased nursing care and monitoring or care

d. The condition is considered to be essential by the family

64. The quality of data is most directly tied to the:

a. Conditions treated in surrounding healthcare settings

b. Surgical case review committee

c. Length of hospital stay

d. Use or application of the data

65. Poor-quality data collection and reporting can affect:

a. Patient care, documentation, revenue generation, outcomes evaluation, and public health reporting

b. Use of patient record for legal purposes

c. Patient care, communication, research activities, and public health reporting

d. Patient care, communication, documentation, revenue generation, outcomes evaluation, research activities, and public health reporting

66. The most succinct definition of where information comes from is:

a. Shredded documents

b. Common blips of data

c. Processed data

d. Measurement of extremities

67. The Joint Commission considers what kind of management to be important for safe, quality care?

a. Resource management

b. Recycling management

c. Information management

d. Incremental management

Domain VI *Information and Communication Technologies*

68. Data warehousing to form clinical repositories is undertaken by merging insurance members' claims and clinical data. Data mining assists in all of the following *except*:

a. Cost cutting

b. Suggest more appropriate medical treatments

c. Providing feedback to patients

d. Predict medical outcomes

69. DRG and APC groupers are usually part of an encoding system in which of the following healthcare settings?

 a. Physician offices

 b. Long-term care facilities

 c. Acute-care hospitals

 d. Outpatient clinics

70. Data, people, and processes along with a combination of hardware, software, and communications technology are components of a(n):

 a. Information system

 b. Classification system

 c. Operating system

 d. Security information

71. Health information exchanges facilitate:

 a. Information system interoperability

 b. Reimbursement processes

 c. Clinician to clinician communication

 d. Seamless transfer of patient care data

72. Digital signatures are:

 a. Methods to detect intrusions

 b. Required for process claims

 c. Cryptography that ensures a document is authentic

 d. A security gateway

73. All of the following are considered malicious software (malware) *except*:

 a. Computer virus

 b. Spyware

 c. Backdoor

 d. Bus typology

74. Clinical information systems are used primarily for:

 a. Patient registration

 b. Admission, discharge, and transfer

 c. Patient care

 d. Clinical document improvement

Domain VII   *Privacy, Confidentiality, Legal, and Ethical Issues*

75. Based on the AHIMA Code of Ethics, which of the following is *not* considered an ethical activity?

    a. Coding audits

    b. Educational purposes within the department

    c. Reviewing the history and physical of a coworker when not part of work assignment

    d. Completion of code assignment

76. Retention policies for the health information department depend on organizational retention policies that must be in accordance with local, state, and federal laws and regulations. These policies vary from institution to institution. In many instances, healthcare institutions may retain health records longer than the law requires. Which of the following statements best describes how the retention of records should be determined?

    a. Unless state or federal law requires longer periods of time, specific patient health information should be retained for established minimum time periods.

    b. AHIMA has published specific guidelines for retention of health information and these guidelines should be followed for records retention.

    c. The Joint Commission has developed standards for retention of health information which must be followed to maintain accreditation and these standards should be adhered to according to these guidelines with regard to time frames.

    d. Health records should be retained according to their use in a facility and the state and federal laws do not apply to the retention of this health information.

77. A patient is admitted to undergo a laparoscopic cholecystectomy. Following the insertion of the laparoscope into the abdominal cavity, the patient experienced a cardiac arrhythmia and the procedure was terminated. The patient experienced a potentially compensable event resulting in an incident report. Which department may request to see the patient's record?

    a. Pediatrics

    b. Risk Management

    c. Surgical Supply

    d. Dietary Services

Domain VIII   *Compliance*

78. Coding compliance policies should include:

    a. Facility-specific documentation requirements

    b. Payer denials

    c. Schedules for record retention

    d. Suggested codes for optimizing reimbursement

79. Under HIPAA Standards for Code Sets, the sets of codes used to encode the diagnoses and procedures, data elements, and medical concepts must be used in:

    a. Paper claims only

    b. Electronic claims only

    c. Outpatient claims only

    d. Inpatient claims only

80. A patient has an inpatient discharge with principal diagnosis of shoulder pain due to peptic ulcer vs. cholecystitis documented on the history and physical. Both are equally treated and well documented. A coder should:

    a. Code whichever diagnosis pays more, if both are equally treated

    b. Use a code from the Findings Abnormal category

    c. Code to the most severe symptom

    d. Code shoulder pain, peptic ulcer, cholecystitis

81. A 75-year-old woman is admitted to the hospital after tripping and falling at home. She underwent an open reduction with internal fixation of the femur. Which of the following would be important to capture in addition to diagnostic codes?

    a. E codes for Cause of Injury and Place of Occurrence

    b. E codes for Cause of Injury, Place of Occurrence, Activity, and Status

    c. E codes for Cause of Injury, Place of Occurrence, and Activity

    d. E codes for Cause of Injury only

Multiple Select Questions

Please select all answers that apply for the following multiple select questions:

82. MS-DRG assignment is based on information that includes _____. (Select all that apply.)

    a. Diagnoses (principal and secondary)

    b. Surgical procedures (principal and secondary)

    c. Diagnostic-related group (DRG) weight

    d. Hospital base rate

    e. Discharge disposition or status

    f. Presence of major or other complications and comorbidities (MCC or CC as secondary diagnosis)

83. The actual payment the hospital is reimbursed is potentially based on all of the following: (Select all that apply.)

    a. If the hospital is an approved teaching hospital

    b. Approved add-on for technology or medical services

    c. Diagnostic-related group (DRG) weight

    d. Hospital base rate

    e. Discharge disposition or status

    f. Disproportionate share hospital adjustment for low-income patients

84. Quality improvement organizations (QIOs) are responsible to which of the following? (Select all that apply.)

    a. Records from hospitals in rural hospitals

    b. Quality of care reviews due to complaints

    c. Utilization Reviews for hospital requested higher weighted DRG payments

    d. Hospital DRG weight review

    e. Review of Emergency Medical Treatment Active Labor Act cases

    f. Disproportionate share hospital adjustment for low income patients

85. Medical necessity is defined by which three factors?

    a. Nonmedical health factors

    b. The likelihood that the service will benefit the patient

    c. Relative value scale

    d. Hospital Base Rate for a diagnosis

    e. Established effectiveness to treat the patient's condition

    f. Procedures are only reimbursed as a covered benefit when performed for a specific diagnosis or specified frequency

86. Assign the correct codes for a total cholecystectomy with exploration of common bile duct and removal of common bile duct stone. (Select all that apply.)

    a. 51.22, Cholecystectomy

    b. 51.23, Laparoscopic cholecystectomy

    c. 51.24, Laparoscopic partial cholecystectomy

    d. 51.41, Common duct exploration for removal of calculus

    e. 51.88, Endoscopic removal of stones from biliary tract

    f. 51.96, Percutaneous extraction of common duct stones

87. Assign the correct codes for a laparoscopic cholecystectomy with percutaneous removal of common bile duct stones. (Select all that apply.)

    a. 47.11, Laparoscopic appendectomy

    b. 51.21, Other partial cholecystectomy

    c. 51.22, Cholecystectomy

    d. 51.23, Laparoscopic cholecystectomy

    e. 51.24, Laparoscopic partial cholecystectomy

    f. 51.41, Common duct exploration for removal of calculus

    g. 51.88, Endoscopic removal of stones from biliary tract

    h. 51.96, Percutaneous extraction of common duct stones

88. Assign the correct codes for a total cholecystectomy with intraoperative cholangiogram and incidental appendectomy. (Select all that apply.)

    a. 47.11, Laparoscopic appendectomy

    b. 47.19, Other incidental appendectomy

    c. 51.21, Other partial cholecystectomy

    d. 51.22, Cholecystectomy

    e. 51.23, Laparoscopic cholecystectomy

    f. 51.24, Laparoscopic partial cholecystectomy

    g. 51.41, Common duct exploration for removal of calculus

    h. 87.53, Intraoperative cholangiogram

89. The convention "omit code" is found only in volume three and usually applies to which of the following? (Select all answers that apply.)

    a. An exploratory procedure incidental to the procedure carried out

    b. 47.19, Other incidental appendectomy

    c. The usual surgical approaches of a given procedure

    d. 51.22, Cholecystectomy

    e. Blunt, digital, manual, or mechanical lysis of adhesions

    f. The closure portion of a procedure

1.	24.	47.	70.
2.	25.	48.	71.
3.	26.	49.	72.
4.	27.	50.	73.
5.	28.	51.	74.
6.	29.	52.	75.
7.	30.	53.	76.
8.	31.	54.	77.
9.	32.	55.	78.
10.	33.	56.	79.
11.	34.	57.	80.
12.	35.	58.	81.
13.	36.	59.	82.
14.	37.	60.	83.
15.	38.	61.	84.
16.	39.	62.	85.
17.	40.	63.	86.
18.	41.	64.	87.
19.	42.	65.	88.
20.	43.	66.	89.
21.	44.	67.	
22.	45.	68.	
23.	46.	69.	

PRACTICE EXAM 1
CASE STUDIES

*Note: Review the Procedures for Coding Medical Record Cases
for the CCS Examination in the Introduction of this book.*

SAME DAY SURGERY SUMMARY—PATIENT 1

HISTORY AND PHYSICAL EXAMINATION

REASON FOR ADMISSION: Breast mass

HISTORY OF PRESENT ILLNESS: The patient is a 57-year-old woman who had a routine mammogram performed last week. A lump was noted on the mammogram about 1.2 cm in size. The patient was referred to me. After an explanation to the patient about the condition, a needle localization breast biopsy was performed which revealed intraductal carcinoma in situ.

PAST MEDICAL HISTORY: Noncontributory

ALLERGIES: None known

CHRONIC MEDICATIONS: None

SOCIAL HISTORY: The patient is a 57-year-old female who is married and lives with her husband. She is a nondrinker and a nonsmoker.

REVIEW OF SYSTEMS: The patient has normal bowels. There is no hematuria or dysuria. The patient has had two colds in the past 6 weeks. She states that she has been having some difficulty sleeping because of worry over this beast mass.

PHYSICAL EXAMINATION: This is a well-developed, well-nourished 57-year-old female who appears younger than her stated age.

 HEENT: PERRLA with supple neck

 LUNGS: The lungs are clear to percussion and auscultation.

 CHEST: The heart has normal rhythm and pulse. There is a mass in the right breast.

 ABDOMEN: Abdomen reveals no masses; bowel sounds are heard.

 EXTREMITIES: Extremities reveal no edema.

IMPRESSION: Intraductal carcinoma right breast

PLAN: The patient came back to the office yesterday morning with her husband. The situation was explained to them. Since this is an intraductal carcinoma in situ. Lumpectomy will be performed and sentinel node dissection will be carried out. Whether the patient needs further treatment or not depends on the findings of the permanent sections of the specimen. The patient and her husband understand the situation very well and agreed to proceed with surgery.

OPERATIVE REPORT—PATIENT 1

PREOPERATIVE DIAGNOSIS: Intraductal carcinoma in situ, right breast, status post biopsy

POSTOPERATIVE DIAGNOSIS: Intraductal carcinoma in situ, right breast, status post biopsy

OPERATION: Lumpectomy and sentinel axillary lymph node dissection

ANESTHESIA: General anesthesia with laryngeal intubation

OPERATIVE REPORT—PATIENT 1 (continued)

PROCEDURE: After obtaining the informed consent, the patient was brought into the operating room and placed on the table in the supine position. General anesthesia with laryngeal intubation was conducted smoothly. The skin over the right chest and right arm was prepped and draped in the usual sterile manner. The intended incision line was marked with a marking pen. The radioactive isotope for the sentinel node dissection was injected. The breast tissue was massaged. Five minutes were then allowed to pass before the incision was made.

The incision was made with excision of the previous incisional scar. The lymphatics were identified and dissected. The suspicious axillary sentinel nodes were dissected. Then the lumpectomy was performed with upper and lower skin flaps. The dissection of the breast tissue and subcutaneous tissue to raise the two flaps was conducted smoothly. A large lump was dissected and the dissection carried to the pectoralis muscles. The big lump was removed completely. Hemostasis was confirmed by cauterization. The wound was then irrigated with copious amounts of warm water solution. The specimen was sent to pathology and the sentinel nodes were sent separately to pathology. The wound was then closed in layers using 2-0 Vicryl for the deeper layer, 3-0 Vicryl for the subcutaneous tissue, and 4-0 Vicryl for the skin.

The patient tolerated the whole procedure very well and was sent to the recovery room in stable condition after extubation.

Blood loss was minimal. Sponge and needle counts were correct. No drain was left. The specimens were sent to pathology.

PATHOLOGY REPORT—PATIENT 1

DATE: 8/3

SPECIMEN: Breast lump and lymph node

GROSS DESCRIPTION: The specimen is submitted as breast and lymphatic tissue. It consists of breast tissue measuring 2.0 cm, 1.5 cm, 1.0 cm.

DIAGNOSIS: Intraductal carcinoma in situ

Enter one diagnosis code and three procedure codes.

PDX

PP1

PR2

PR3

SAME-DAY SURGERY SUMMARY — PATIENT 2

DATE OF ADMISSION: 8/3   **DATE OF DISCHARGE:** 8/3

DISCHARGE DIAGNOSIS:

1. Sinus infection

2. Chronic otitis media

3. Adenoid hypertrophy

PROCEDURES:

1. Adenoidectomy

2. Bilateral myringotomy

INSTRUCTIONS ON DISCHARGE:

Contact my office for follow-up in 1 week

Take Augmentin 500 mg by mouth BID per day for 10 days

Darvocet 1 tablet every 4 hours for pain as needed

HISTORY AND PHYSICAL EXAMINATION — PATIENT 2

ADMITTED: 8/3

REASON FOR ADMISSION: This is a 35-year-old patient who has recurrent sinusitis and chronic otitis media. The patient also suffers from adenoidal obstruction of the eustachian tubes and nasopharynx. Treatment has consisted of antihistamines and decongestants as well as antibiotic therapy. This has been ineffective to control the inflammation. The patient has requested surgery for definitive treatment of the condition.

PAST MEDICAL HISTORY: Negative

ALLERGIES: None known

CHRONIC MEDICATIONS: None

FAMILY HISTORY: Noncontributory

REVIEW OF SYSTEMS: The patient has had repeated office visits over the past 3 years for sinusitis and otitis media. The patient has no other health problems.

PHYSICAL EXAMINATION: This is a Hispanic female in no acute distress. BP is 120/70. Temp. is 99.0 degrees. Pulse is 72. Respirations 12.

    HEENT: Tympanic membranes are red with perforation of the tympanic membrane and hearing loss. Otherwise normal.

    NECK: Supple

    CHEST: Clear to percussion and auscultation

    HEART: Regular force, rate, and rhythm

    ABDOMINAL: Normal, no masses

    EXTREMITIES: No edema, normal

IMPRESSION: Sinus infection and chronic otitis media

PROGRESS NOTES—PATIENT 2

DATE   **NOTE**

8/3   Patient is alert and oriented. Admitted to Same-Day Surgery for adenoidectomy and insertion of myringotomy tubes.

PREOPERATIVE DIAGNOSIS:

Chronic sinusitis

POSTOPERATIVE DIAGNOSIS:

1. Chronic sinusitis

2. Otitis media; Adenoid obstruction of the eustachian tube and nasopharynx

OPERATION:

Bilateral myringotomy with insertion of Shepard tympanostomy tubes; Adenoidectomy

ANESTHESIA: General

COMPLICATIONS: None

The patient tolerated the procedure well. No bleeding noted. Will discharge patient when transportation available.

PHYSICIAN'S ORDERS—PATIENT 2

DATE   **ORDER**

8/3   Patient is admitted for adenoidectomy and myringotomy

Prep patient for surgery

NPO

PREOP ORDERS

Morphine 10 mg IM upon admission

Atropine 0.4 mg IM upon admission

POSTOP ORDERS

Ice collar

T & A Precautions

OOB ad lib

Darvocet-N tabs, one every 4 hours p.r.n. pain

Demerol 75 mg PO now

Discharge after 4:00 p.m. when stable

OPERATIVE REPORT—PATIENT 2

DATE: 8/3

PREOPERATIVE DIAGNOSIS: Chronic sinusitis, otitis media, adenoid obstruction of the eustachian tubes and nasopharynx

POSTOPERATIVE DIAGNOSIS: Chronic sinusitis, serous otitis media, adenoid obstruction of the eustachian tubes and nasopharynx

OPERATION: Bilateral myringotomy with insertion of Shepard tympanostomy tubes; Adenoidectomy

ANESTHESIA: General

OPERATIVE PROCEDURE: Following the induction of general anesthesia, patient was prepped and draped in the usual sterile manner for the above mentioned procedures. The left ear was approached first.

The tympanic membrane was found to be injected, retracted, and full of a serous fluid. An anterior myringotomy incision was performed, and a Shepard tympanostomy tube was inserted in place.

Following this, an identical procedure was done on the right side, except on the right side the fluid was gray and viscous, and the tympanic membrane had already developed tympanosclerotic scar tissue throughout the tympanic membrane. An anterior myringotomy incision was performed, and a Shepard tympanostomy tube was inserted in place.

Following this, the patient was prepared and draped in the usual manner for adenoidectomy. With the soft palate retracted, an adenoid mass filling the entire nasopharynx was visualized. It was removed with adenoid curettes until the normal anatomical structures of the torus tubarius and the posterior choanae of the nasal passages could clearly be seen. The adenoid tissue trailed into the nose and into the area of the infundibulum of the middle meatus. Hemostasis was achieved.

The patient was awakened from anesthesia and taken to the recovery room in good condition.

PATHOLOGY REPORT — PATIENT 2

DATE: 8/3

SPECIMEN: Adenoids

GROSS DESCRIPTION: The specimen is submitted as adenoids. It consists of multiple fragments of adenoid tissue, the largest measuring 2.5 cm, 1.5 cm, 1.0 cm. These fragments are similar to tonsillar tissues.

MICROSCOPIC DESCRIPTION: There are no significant pathologic lesions seen grossly.

DIAGNOSIS: Adenoids

Enter three diagnosis codes and two procedure codes.

PDX

DX2

DX3

PP1

PR2

SAME-DAY SURGERY SUMMARY — PATIENT 3

HISTORY AND PHYSICAL EXAMINATION

DATE: 1/29

HISTORY OF PRESENT ILLNESS: This is a 62-year-old male with progressive painful blurring of vision due to aphakic bullous keratopathy with glaucoma. He has undergone previous Molteno implant with poor vision and pain due to ruptured bulla. The patient is admitted for transplant, vitrectomy and lens implantation at this time.

PAST MEDICAL HISTORY: The patient has angina and COPD. There have been no recent episodes of chest pain or shortness of breath. The patient also underwent a prostatectomy six years ago for prostatic carcinoma.

ALLERGIES: None known

CHRONIC MEDICATIONS: Ventolin and nitroglycerin as needed for chest pain

SOCIAL HISTORY: The patient is a 62-year-old male who is married and lives with his wife. He has 5 grandchildren. He is a nondrinker and a nonsmoker.

REVIEW OF SYSTEMS: The patient has normal bowels. He has had no problems with his urine since his prostatectomy. There is no hematuria or dysuria. The patient has had two colds in the past six weeks. He states that he has been having some difficulty sleeping because of the pain in his shoulder. This has limited some of the activity that he normally does, such as golf.

PHYSICAL EXAMINATION: This is a well-developed, well-nourished 62-year-old male who appears younger than his stated age.

HEENT: Aphakic, neck supple

CHEST: The lungs are clear to percussion and auscultation. The heart has normal rhythm and pulse.

ABDOMEN: Abdomen reveals no masses; bowel sounds are heard.

EXTREMITIES: Extremities reveal no edema.

OPERATIVE REPORT — PATIENT 3

PREOPERATIVE DIAGNOSES:

1. Aphakic bullous keratopathy

2. Open-angle glaucoma

3. Chronic iritis

POSTOPERATIVE DIAGNOSES:

1. Aphakic bullous keratopathy

2. Open-angle glaucoma

3. Chronic iritis

OPERATION:

1. Aphakic penetrating keratoplasty

2. Posterior chamber intraocular lens scleral implant

3. Open-sky mechanical automated vitrectomy

ANESTHESIA: Retrobulbar block, monitored anesthesia care

COMPLICATIONS: None

INDICATIONS: This is a 62-year-old gentleman with progressive painful blurring of vision due to aphakic bullous keratopathy with glaucoma. He has undergone previous Molteno implant with poor vision and pain due to ruptured bulla. The patient is admitted for transplant vitrectomy and lens implantation of the left eye at this time. After informed consent, the patient agreed to the benefits and risks of surgery.

PROCEDURE DESCRIPTION: The patient was taken to the operating room. Under monitored anesthesia care, he was given a retrobulbar block in the standard fashion for a total of 4 cc of a 50/50 mixture 0.75% Marcaine and 4% lidocaine with Wydase.

After ensuring adequate anesthesia as well as akinesia, the patient was prepped and draped in the usual sterile ophthalmologic fashion. A wire lid speculum was inserted, and a small conjunctival peritomy was made at the two o'clock and ten o'clock hour positions to prepare for half-thickness scleral flaps for suturing a scleral-supported lens in the left eye. A Flieringa ring was then attached in the standard fashion using four interrupted 5-0 Dacron sutures. Attention was then placed to the back Mayo, and a 7.75-mm donor button was harvested, epithelial side down, in the standard fashion. Routine surveillance cultures were sent, and the donor button was placed on the Mayo stand in a Petri dish. Attention was then placed on the donor's cornea, and using a Barron-Hessburg trephine device, a 7.50-mm button was harvested under viscoelastic support. Corneoscleral scissors were used to the left and right respectively to remove the button in toto. Vitrectomy was then performed due to prolapsing vitreous, and an attempt to reposition the iris was made. However, due to loss of iris material during prior surgeries, I was unable to close the sphincter defect. After completing the vitrectomy, a scleral-supported CZ70VD 7-mm lens was secured using a 10-0 Prolene suture at the ten and two o'clock hour positions. Scleral flaps were then closed over the 10-0 Prolene to maintain a tight closure. The button was then sewn into position using 16 interrupted 10-0 nylon sutures in the standard fashion. All the knots were cut short and buried in the recipient side of the host junction. A final check to make sure the chamber was watertight was unremarkable, and the Flieringa ring was removed followed by the bridle sutures. Subconjunctival Ancef and Celestone were placed, and a bandage contact lens was placed on the eye.

The patient was taken to the recovery room in good repair without complications of the above procedure.

Enter six diagnosis codes and three procedure codes.

PDX

DX2

DX3

DX4

DX5

DX6

PP1

PR2

PR3

Emergency Department E/M Mapping Scenario for Emergency Department Cases 4 and 5

Code the procedures that are done in the emergency department as well as the E/M code derived from the mapping scenario.

Point Value Key

Level 1 = 1–20

Level 2 = 21–35

Level 3 = 36–47

Level 4 = 48–60

Level 5 = > 61

Critical Care > 61 with constant physician attendance

CPT Codes

Level 1   99281   99281–25 with procedure/laboratory/radiology

Level 2   99282   99282–25 with procedure/laboratory/radiology

Level 3   99283   99283–25 with procedure/laboratory/radiology

Level 4   99284   99284–25 with procedure/laboratory/radiology

Level 5   99285   99285–25 with procedure/laboratory/radiology

Emergency Department Acuity Points					
	5	10	15	20	25
Meds Given	1–2	3–5	6–7	8–9	> 10
Extent of Hx	Brief	PF	EPF	Detail	Comprehensive
Extent of Examination	Brief	PF	EPF	Detail	Comprehensive
Number of Tests Ordered	0–1	2–3	4–5	6–7	> 8
Supplies Used	1	2–3	4–5	6–7	> 8

EMERGENCY DEPARTMENT RECORD—PATIENT 4

DATE OF ADMISSION: 4/1   **DATE OF DISCHARGE:** 4/1

HISTORY (Problem Focused):

HISTORY OF PRESENT ILLNESS: This 16-year-old African-American female underwent piercing of her ears. The patient was removing her sweater when she accidentally pulled the earring through her ear lobe.

PAST MEDICAL HISTORY: The patient has a history of childhood asthma that has not occurred for several years.

ALLERGIES: Penicillin

CHRONIC MEDICATIONS: None

REVIEW OF SYSTEMS: The patient has been well.

PHYSICAL EXAMINATION (Problem Focused):

GENERAL APPEARANCE: This is a well-nourished 16-year-old black female in no apparent distress. HEENT normal except for 2 cm laceration of left earlobe. Neck veins flat at 40-degree angle. No nodes felt in the neck, carotids, or groin. Carotid pulsations are normal. No bruits heard in the neck. Chest clear on percussion and auscultation. Heart is not enlarged. No thrills or murmurs. Rhythm is regular. BP 130/80. Liver and spleen not palpable. No masses felt in the abdomen. No ascites noted. No edema of the extremities. Pulses in the feet are good.

IMPRESSION: Laceration of left ear lobe

PLAN: Suture laceration of ear lobe

TREATMENT: Following infiltration of the areas with Xylocaine, the laceration was closed with 2-0 Vicryl. Two suture kits were used.

DISCHARGE DIAGNOSIS: Ear lobe laceration of left ear

INSTRUCTIONS ON DISCHARGE: Demerol by mouth 50 mg every 6 hours as needed for pain. Biaxin 500 mg PO b.i.d. for 10 days. Follow up with surgical clinic in 7 days.

Enter one diagnosis code and two procedure codes.

PDX

PP1

PR2

EMERGENCY DEPARTMENT RECORD—PATIENT 5

DATE OF ADMISSION: 6/17   **DATE OF DISCHARGE:** 6/17

HISTORY (Problem Focused):

ADMISSION HISTORY: This is a 29-year-old Asian female. She was walking down her steps when she fell. The patient complains of pain in the arm.

ALLERGIES: Penicillin

CHRONIC MEDICATIONS: Normally takes no drugs but has been taking ibuprofen every 6 hours because of painful arm.

FAMILY HISTORY: Noncontributory

SOCIAL HISTORY: The patient smokes one pack of cigarettes per day. She drinks one drink per day.

REVIEW OF SYSTEMS: The patient had hives the last time she took penicillin. Her cardiovascular, genitourinary, and gastrointestinal systems are negative.

PHYSICAL EXAMINATION (Expanded Problem Focused):

GENERAL APPEARANCE: This is an alert cooperative female in no acute distress.

HEENT: PERRLA, extraocular movements are full

NECK: Supple

CHEST: Lungs are clear. Heart has normal sinus rhythm.

ABDOMEN: Soft and nontender, no organomegaly

EXTREMITIES: Examination of the arm reveals painful movement.

LABORATORY AND X-RAY DATA: Urinalysis is normal; EKG normal; chest x-ray is normal; CBC and diff show no abnormalities; x-ray of the left arm revealed a fracture of the shaft of the humerus.

IMPRESSION: Fracture of the shaft of the humerus

PLAN: Reduction fracture of the humerus

TREATMENT: Following administration of conscious sedation, the patient's humeral fracture was reduced and a cast applied. One fracture tray was used.

DISCHARGE DIAGNOSIS: Fracture of the left shaft of the humerus

INSTRUCTIONS ON DISCHARGE: The patient is instructed to make an appointment with the orthopedic clinic in 3 days, to take one Percocet every 4 hours as needed for pain as per the label. Call the ER doctor if swelling or blue color of the fingers occurs. The patient is also counseled to stop smoking and was instructed to make an appointment with her primary care physician to discuss smoking cessation.

Enter two diagnosis codes and two procedure codes.

PDX

DX2

PP1

PR2

AMBULATORY RECORD—PATIENT 6

Right and left heart catheterization and coronary angiography

PROCEDURE: After obtaining informed consent the patient was taken to the cardiac catheterization laboratory. The right groin was prepped and draped in the usual fashion and 2% Xylocaine was used to anesthetize. 6-French sheaths were introduced into the right femoral artery and vein and a 6-French multipurpose catheter was used for the heart catheterization, coronary angiography, and ventricular angiography. Right heart pressures and cardiac outputs were measured. A pigtail catheter was inserted into the left ventricular cavity and ventricular pressures obtained. Angiography of the right coronary artery was performed. Left ventricular angiography and aortic root angiography was performed. The patient tolerated the procedure well without complications.

DIAGNOSIS: Arteriosclerotic coronary artery disease

Enter one diagnosis code and two procedure codes.

PDX

PP1

PR2

INTERVENTIONAL RADIOLOGY REPORT — PATIENT 7

EXAMINATION: Ultrasound guided liver biopsy

HISTORY: Carcinoma of the lower right lobe of the lung

PROCEDURE: Limited real-time transabdominal ultrasound of the liver was performed. There is a 3.5 × 2.9-cm mass in the lateral segment of the left lobe of the liver. This mass is hypoechogenic with increased blood flow. Following informed consent the patient was prepped and draped in the usual manner. Using ultrasound guidance, percutaneous fine-needle aspiration biopsy of the left lobe of the liver mass was performed. The patient tolerated the procedure well.

IMPRESSION: Hypoechogenic mass in the left lobe of the liver that was successfully biopsied with ultrasound guidance

PATHOLOGY REPORT: Metastatic lung carcinoma

Enter two diagnosis codes and two procedure codes.

PDX

DX2

PP1

PR2

INPATIENT RECORD — PATIENT 8

DISCHARGE SUMMARY

DATE OF ADMISSION: 11/30   **DATE OF DISCHARGE:** 12/4

DISCHARGE DIAGNOSIS: Fractured neck of right femur

ADMISSION HISTORY: The patient is a 78-year-old male who fell on the day of admission and sustained a fracture of the neck of his right femur. The patient was admitted for a medical evaluation prior to surgical intervention.

COURSE IN HOSPITAL: Medical evaluation was obtained on admission. Patient was taken to the operating room, where an open reduction and internal fixation of the fracture of the right femur was performed. Postoperative course was unremarkable except for urinary retention, which necessitated the placement of an indwelling Foley catheter. He was discharged with the catheter in place. The patient was ambulatory, nonweight bearing with a walker at the time of discharge.

INSTRUCTIONS ON DISCHARGE: The patient is instructed to follow up with my office in 3 days to remove staples and to begin outpatient physical therapy tomorrow. Home health services will follow this patient. Pain medications: Darvocet N 100, one tablet every 4 hours as needed for pain.

HISTORY AND PHYSICAL EXAMINATION — PATIENT 8

ADMITTED: 11/30

REASON FOR ADMISSION: Right hip pain following a fall

HISTORY OF PRESENT ILLNESS: The patient is a 78-year-old male who fell on the day of admission and sustained a fracture of the neck of his right femur. The patient was admitted for a medical evaluation prior to surgical intervention.

PAST MEDICAL HISTORY: The patient has had multiple medical problems including gastric ulcer, congestive heart failure, diverticulosis, degenerative joint disease, arteriosclerotic coronary artery disease, and mitral regurgitation.

ALLERGIES: None

CHRONIC MEDICATIONS: Lanoxin 0.125 mg, Mon. Wed., and Fri., Lasix 40 mg q. a.m., Lasix 40 mg q. p.m., Colace 200 mg q. a.m., Metamucil one teaspoon b.i.d., Zestril 10 mg every day, Zantac 150 mg PO b.i.d., nitroglycerin 0.4 mg. PRN for chest pain, Celebrex 100 mg PO b.i.d. for degenerative joint disease.

SOCIAL HISTORY: The patient is widowed with 3 children and 7 grandchildren. The patient is a nondrinker and nonsmoker.

REVIEW OF SYSTEMS: The patient has been in usual health until the day prior to admission when he fell. There has been no change in bladder and bowel functioning. Cognitively, he has experienced some confusion on and off lately.

PHYSICAL EXAMINATION: BP is 170/90, pulse 80 and regular. The patient is an elderly, thin, somewhat deaf male. His pupils are small and reactive to light. The pharynx is benign. The jugular pulse is distended but filled from above. He has no supraclavicular adenopathy. His chest is clear. On palpation the pericardium was located in his anterior axillary line with a palpable thrill. On auscultation he had a harsh grade III/VI apical systolic murmur that radiated to the apex and faintly to the lower left sternal edge. He had a soft diastolic flow murmur. His abdomen was somewhat tense without organomegaly. He had minimal peripheral edema.

CONSULTATION—PATIENT 8

DATE: 11/30

CHIEF COMPLAINT: Pain in hip

REVIEW OF SYSTEMS: The patient has been in usual health until the day prior to admission when he fell. The patient is experiencing a little more shortness of breath than usual. The patient is unsure if he felt dizzy before falling.

PHYSICAL EXAMINATION: This is an elderly, moderately nourished white male. HEENT reveals nothing abnormal. There is no adenopathy. His chest is clear with loud grade III/VI pansystolic murmur. Examination of the abdomen reveals no masses or tenderness. He had minimal peripheral edema with one leg appearing shorter than the other. Distal circulation and sensation are normal.

IMPRESSION:

History of gastric ulcer

Congestive heart failure

Diverticulosis

Degenerative joint disease

Arteriosclerotic coronary artery disease

Mitral regurgitation

PLAN: D/C NSAIDs for now in light of GI history. The patient is cleared for surgery.

PROGRESS NOTES—PATIENT 8

DATE	NOTE
11/30	Patient admitted for medical evaluation prior to ORIF. The patient is somewhat confused about the events surrounding the fall. At present he offers no other complaint. The patient currently has Bucks traction in place. If cleared for surgery, patient is scheduled for tomorrow at 1:00 p.m.
12/1	The patient is resting quietly. Medication adequate to alleviate pain in extremity.
6:30 a.m.	Operative consent signed following obtaining informed consent for surgery. All questions from patient and family answered. **PREOP DX:** Fracture of right femur
6:30 p.m.	**POSTOP DX:** Same **OPERATION:** Open reduction, internal fixation, fracture, right hip **ANESTHESIA:** Spinal and general **COMPLICATIONS:** None Patient sleeping. Dressings intact, hemovac in place.
8:00 p.m.	House Physician called to see patient due to inability to void. The patient appears to have postop urinary retention. Will place Foley catheter.
12/2	Events of last night noted. Will request that patient get OOB and begin physical therapy. Hemovac in place draining small amount. Patient not complaining of pain. H&H looks good. Lytes fine.
12/3	Patient has been ambulating well. Patient minimally confused due to senile dementia. Neurovascular status good. Appetite good. Dressing intact, incision healing well, no redness or inflammation.
12/4	Patient up with assistance and ambulating using walker. Incision healing well. Discharge with indwelling Foley. Home health services to assist patient following discharge. Ready for discharge today.

PHYSICIAN'S ORDERS—PATIENT 8

DATE	ORDER
11/30	Admit to floor
	NPO after midnight
	Continue present meds:
	Lanoxin 0.125 mg, q.d.
	Lasix 40 mg q. a.m. and p.m.
	Colace 200 mg q. a.m.
	Metamucil one teaspoon b.i.d.
	Zantac 150 mg po b.i.d.
	Celebrex 100 mg po b.i.d. for DJD
	Prep for hip surgery
	Medical Consult for surgical clearance
	4 lb Bucks traction to continue
	Demerol 50 mg q. 3 to 4 hours
	Darvocet N 100 q. 3 to 4 hours
	Cross match 3 units of blood
	Low sodium, low-fat diet
	Dig level in a.m.
	H&H and electrolytes
12/1	Preop Meds
	Hold Dig this a.m.
	Ancef 1 g on call to OR
	Postop Meds
	Run D5W 1,000 cc q. 12 hrs
	Demerol 500 mg q. 3 to 4 hrs p.r.n. pain
	Darvocet N 100 q. 3 to 4 hours
	Hct and Hgb at 9:00 p.m. and in a.m.
	Electrolytes in a.m.
	Ancef 500 mg IV q. 6 hrs ×4 doses
	X-ray hip in a.m.
	Ice on hip
	Up in chair following x-ray
	Begin physical therapy tomorrow
	Insert Foley catheter
12/2	Consult home health services for discharge needs. Continue pain meds. Get patient OOB for ambulation with walker.
12/3	D/C IV
12/4	D/C patient. Home health services to follow.

OPERATIVE REPORT—PATIENT 8

DATE: 12/1

PREOPERATIVE DIAGNOSIS: Fracture of right femur

POSTOPERATIVE DIAGNOSIS: Same

OPERATION: Open reduction and internal fixation of fracture right hip

ANESTHESIA: Spinal and general

OPERATIVE INDICATIONS:

OPERATIVE PROCEDURE: The patient was given Ancef 1 g IV 30 minutes prior to the procedure for endocarditis/ surgical prophylaxis. The patient was administered a spinal anesthesia and then placed on the fracture table in traction. X-rays revealed satisfactory position and alignment of the fracture site. The right hip was prepped with Betadine scrub and Betadine solution and draped in a sterile fashion. A straight incision was made over the lateral aspect of the right hip and carried through the subcutaneous tissue, then tensor fascia lata and vastus lateralis muscles so that the fracture could be reduced and fixation devices utilized. The lateral shaft of the femur was exposed subperiosteally. A guide wire was then placed into the neck and head of the femur and x-rays revealed a slightly inferior position. The new guide wire was obtained in satisfactory position. The lateral shaft, neck, and head of the femur were then drilled to a depth of 85 mm with the drill. An 85-mm, 140-degree and 5-degree compression nail were then inserted over which a 140-degree angle 4-hole side plate was then inserted. A compression screw was then applied after the key was inserted. The side plate was then fixed to the shaft of the femur with four screws. X-rays revealed satisfactory position and alignment of the fracture fragments and the fixation device. The wound was then well irrigated. A large hemovac drain was inserted and brought out through a separate stab wound incision. The wound was closed with a continuous #000 Vicryl suture in the vastus lateralis and tensor fascia lata layers. The subcutaneous tissue was closed with interrupted #000 Vicryl sutures and the skin was closed with staples. A compression dressing was applied. The patient tolerated the procedure well and there were no operative complications. Patient was returned to the recovery room in satisfactory condition.

LABORATORY REPORTS—PATIENT 8

HEMATOLOGY

DATE: 11/30

Specimen	Results	Normal Values
WBC	9.9	4.3–11.0
RBC	5.0	4.5–5.9
HGB	14.0	13.5–17.5
HCT	45	41–52
MCV	89	80–100
MCHC	33.9	31–57
PLT	Adequate	150–450

HEMATOLOGY—PATIENT 8

DATE: 12/1

Specimen	Results	Normal Values
WBC	7.7	4.3–11.0
RBC	4.4 L	4.5–5.9
HGB	13.2 L	13.5–17.5
HCT	41	41–52
MCV	89	80–100
MCHC	33.9	31–57
PLT	Adequate	150–450

HEMATOLOGY—PATIENT 8

DATE: 12/1

Specimen	Results	Normal Values
WBC	8.0	4.3–11.0
RBC	4.5	4.5–5.9
HGB	13.7	13.5–17.5
HCT	42	41–52
MCV	89	80–100
MCHC	33.9	31–57
PLT	Adequate	150–450

LABORATORY REPORTS — PATIENT 8 (continued)

CHEMISTRY—PATIENT 8

DATE: 11/30

Specimen	Results	Normal Values
GLUC	97	70–110
BUN	12	8–25
CREAT	1.0	0.5–1.5
NA	138	136–146
K	4.0	3.5–5.5
CL	109	95–110
CO_2	33 H	24–32
CA	9.1	8.4–10.5
PHOS	3.0	2.5–4.4
MG	2.0	1.6–3.0
T BILI	1.0	0.2–1.2
D BILI	0.4	0.0–0.5
PROTEIN	7.0	6.0–8.0
ALBUMIN	5.4	5.0–5.5
AST	36	0–40
ALT	44	30–65
GCT	70	15–85
LD	110	100–190
ALK PHOS	114	50–136
URIC ACID	6.0	2.2–7.7
CHOL	165	0–200
TRIG	140	10–160

LABORATORY REPORTS — PATIENT 8 *(continued)*

CHEMISTRY—PATIENT 8

DATE: 12/1

Specimen	Results	Normal Values
GLUC	97	70–110
BUN	12	8–25
CREAT	1.0	0.5–1.5
NA	134 L	136–146
K	5.6 H	3.5–5.5
CL	109	95–110
CO_2	33 H	24–32
CA	9.1	8.4–10.5
PHOS	3.0	2.5–4.4
MG	2.0	1.6–3.0
T BILI	1.0	0.2–1.2
D BILI	0.4	0.0–0.5
PROTEIN	7.0	6.0–8.0
ALBUMIN	5.4	5.0–5.5
AST	36	0–40
ALT	44	30–65
GGT	70	15–85
LD	110	100–190
ALK PHOS	114	50–136
URIC ACID	6.0	2.2–7.7
CHOL	165	0–200
TRIG	140	10–160

RADIOLOGY REPORT — PATIENT 8

DATE: 11/30

RIGHT HIP AND FEMUR: A displaced intertrochanteric fracture is noted with a mild degree of varus angulation. The adjacent skeletal structures are normal. The right femur is intact beyond the hip. There is vascular calcification.

CHEST, SUPINE: There is no gross evidence of acute inflammatory disease or congestive heart failure.

IMPRESSION: Femur and hip; slightly angulated intertrochanteric fracture; chest; no acute disease.

RADIOLOGY REPORT — PATIENT 8

DATE: 12/2

DIAGNOSIS: RIGHT HIP AND FEMUR. The displaced intertrochanteric fracture has been surgically corrected. The adjacent skeletal structures are normal.

IMPRESSION: The fracture is maintained with an orthopedic device.

Enter ten diagnosis codes and one procedure code.

PDX

DX2

DX3

DX4

DX5

DX6

DX7

DX8

DX9

DX10

PP1

INPATIENT RECORD—PATIENT 9

DISCHARGE SUMMARY

DATE OF ADMISSION: 2/3   **DATE OF DISCHARGE:** 2/5

DISCHARGE DIAGNOSIS: Full-term pregnancy—delivered male infant

Patient started labor spontaneously three days before her due date. She was brought to the hospital by automobile. Labor progressed for a while but then contractions became fewer and she delivered soon after. A midline episiotomy was done. Membranes and placenta were complete. There was some bleeding but not excessive. Patient made an uneventful recovery.

HISTORY AND PHYSICAL EXAMINATION—PATIENT 9

ADMITTED: 2/3

REASON FOR ADMISSION: Full-term pregnancy

PAST MEDICAL HISTORY: Previous deliveries normal and mitral valve prolapse

ALLERGIES: None known

CHRONIC MEDICATIONS: None

FAMILY HISTORY: Heart disease—father

SOCIAL HISTORY: The patient is married and has one other child living with her.

REVIEW OF SYSTEMS:

   SKIN: Normal

   HEAD-SCALP: Normal

   EYES: Normal

   ENT: Normal

   NECK: Normal

   BREASTS: Normal

   THORAX: Normal

   LUNGS: Normal

   HEART: Slight midsystolic click with late systolic murmur II/VI

   ABDOMEN: Normal

IMPRESSION: Good health with term pregnancy. History of mitral valve prolapse—asymptomatic.

PROGRESS NOTES—PATIENT 9

DATE	NOTE
2/3	Admit to Labor and Delivery. MVP stable. Patient progressing well. Delivered at 1:15 p.m. one full-term male infant.
2/4	Patient doing well. Mitral valve prolapse stable. The perineum is clean and dry, incision intact.
2/5	Will discharge to home

PHYSICIAN'S ORDERS—PATIENT 9

DATE	ORDER
2/3	Admit to Labor and Delivery 1,000 cc 5% D/LR May ambulate Type and screen CBC May have ice chips
2/5	Discharge patient to home.

DELIVERY RECORD—PATIENT 9

DATE: 2/3

The patient was 3 cm dilated when admitted. The duration of the first stage of labor was 6 hours, second stage was 14 minutes, third stage was 5 minutes. She was given local anesthesia. An episiotomy was performed with repair. There were no lacerations. The cord was wrapped once around the baby's neck, but did not cause compression. The mother and liveborn baby were discharged from the delivery room in good condition.

LABORATORY REPORT — PATIENT 9

HEMATOLOGY

DATE: 2/3

Specimen	Results	Normal Values
WBC	5.2	4.3–11.0
RBC	4.9	4.5–5.9
HGB	13.8	13.5–17.5
HCT	45	41–52
MCV	93	80–100
MCHC	41	31–57
PLT	255	150–450

Enter four diagnosis codes and one procedure code.

PDX

DX2

DX3

DX4

PP1

INPATIENT RECORD—PATIENT 10

DISCHARGE SUMMARY

DATE OF ADMISSION: 1/31   **DATE OF DISCHARGE:** 2/3

DISCHARGE DIAGNOSIS: Right lower lobe pneumonia due to gram-negative bacteria, resistant to erythromycin

ADMISSION HISTORY: This is a 56-year-old insulin-requiring diabetic female whose diabetes is out of control whom we have been following for hypertension, degenerative joint disease, aortic stenosis and diabetic retinopathy. Over the past three days she has noted increased cough and chest congestion with a fever of approximately 102 degrees. She was found to have a right lower lobe infiltrate and was started on therapy with erythromycin. Despite initial therapy, the patient's clinical status has worsened over the past 24 hours.

COURSE IN HOSPITAL: Patient was admitted with the diagnosis of right lower lobe pneumonia. She was begun on intravenous ceftriaxone. Because of difficulties with venous access, patient was switched to intramuscular ceftriaxone on her third hospital day.

By 2/3 the patient was afebrile and her cough had diminished. Her blood pressure was well controlled at 140/74.

INSTRUCTIONS ON DISCHARGE: Follow up with me by phone in three days and in my office in two weeks. Repeat chest x-ray to be done then.

MEDICATIONS:

1. Calan SR 180 mg b.i.d.
2. Zestril 20 mg PO q. a.m.
3. NPH Insulin, 30 units, sub q., a.m.
4. Levoquin 500 mg PO daily ×10 days
5. Celebrex 100 mg PO b.i.d.

HISTORY AND PHYSICAL EXAMINATION—PATIENT 10

ADMITTED: 1/31

REASON FOR ADMISSION: Physical examination on admission revealed a well-developed, acutely ill-appearing black female.

HISTORY OF PRESENT ILLNESS: A 56-year-old diabetic followed for hypertension and diabetic retinopathy. Over the past three days she has noted increased cough and chest congestion with a fever of approximately 102 degrees. She was found to have a right lower lobe infiltrate and was begun on therapy with erythromycin. Despite initial therapy, the patient's clinical status worsened over the past 24 hours and hospitalization was recommended.

PAST MEDICAL HISTORY: Hypertension, degenerative joint disease in both knees, and moderate aortic stenosis

ALLERGIES: Dust

CHRONIC MEDICATIONS: CalanSR 180 mg po b.i.d., Insulin (NPH), Zestril 20 mg PO daily, Celebrex 100 mg PO b.i.d.

FAMILY HISTORY: Notable for hypertension in mother

SOCIAL HISTORY: Noncontributory

PHYSICAL EXAMINATION:

    GENERAL APPEARANCE: The patient is a well-developed black female in moderate distress.

    VITAL SIGNS: T 102, P 80, R 16, BP 150/80

    SKIN: Warm and dry

    HEENT: Significant for mildly inflamed mucous membranes. Retinopathy evident in both eyes.

    NECK: Supple. Symmetrical with no bruits

    LUNGS: Coarse rhonchi bilaterally, right greater than left

    HEART: Regular rate and rhythm, positive S1, positive III/VI SEM

    ABDOMEN: Soft, nontender, no mass

GENITALIA: Deferred

RECTAL: Deferred

EXTREMITIES: No edema

NEUROLOGIC: Normal

HISTORY AND PHYSICAL EXAMINATION—PATIENT 10

LABORATORY DATA:

1. EKG: NSR, widespread ST-T wave abnormalities, LV hypertrophy

2. CBC: Hgb 13, Hct 38, WBC 12.8

3. Glucose: 281

4. Urinalysis: Unremarkable

5. Sputum: Gram stain—a few WBCs, moderate gram-negative rods

IMPRESSION:

1. Right lower lobe pneumonia possibly due to gram-negative bacteria

2. Diabetes mellitus on insulin—uncontrolled

3. Hypertension—stable

4. Degenerative joint disease—stable

5. Moderate aortic stenosis

PLAN: Admit, IV antibiotics for pneumonia. Monitor blood sugars.

PROGRESS NOTES—PATIENT 10

DATE	NOTE
1/31	Patient admitted for cough associated with increased temperature with chest x-ray indicative of pneumonia. Will obtain sputum culture and begin on ceftriaxone. Will monitor blood pressure and blood sugars. Will use sliding scale to bring blood sugar into control. Patient with recent echocardiogram as outpatient that showed stable aortic stenosis.
2/1	The patient is responding well. Will request diabetic education nurse to meet with her and set up an appointment for classes following this admission.
2/2	Sputum culture reveals gram-negative bacteria as suspected. Patient's temperature is down. Patient resting comfortably. Blood sugar better.
2/3	Blood sugar with increasing control today. The importance of appropriate diet emphasized. Will discharge with p.o. antibiotics.

PHYSICIAN'S ORDERS — PATIENT 10

DATE	ORDER
1/31/20XX	Admit to 3 South
	DX: Pneumonia
	Please give ceftriaxone 1 g q 8 hours IV
	ADA diet
	CBC and SMA
	CalanSR 50 mg in a.m. with orange juice
	Zestril 2 in a.m.
	Celebrex 100 mg po BID
	Accucheck before meals and before bedtime
	Chest x-ray
	Sliding scale for insulin as follows:
	Below 120 give 4 units of regular
	120–200 give 6 units of regular insulin
	200–300 give 8 units of regular insulin
	Above 300, call physician
2/1/20XX	Change insulin to 40 NPH units sq in a.m. today.
	Consult diabetic nurse to see patient and set up classes following admission.
2/2/20XX	Continue insulin to 40 NPH units sq in a.m. today.
2/2/20XX	D/C IV and switch to ceftriaxone 1 g IM q. 24 hrs
2/3/20XX	Discharge to home.

LABORATORY REPORTS—PATIENT 10

MICROBIOLOGY

DATE   **TEST TYPE**

1/31/20XX SOURCE:
SITE:
GRAM STAIN RESULTS: Sputum
CULTURE RESULTS: Slight WBCs, Slight Epis
Many gram-negative rods
sl. gram-negative diplococci
sl. gram-positive cocci in clusters

SUSCEPTIBILITY:	S
AMPICILLIN	S
CEFAZOLIN	S
CEFOTAXIME	S
CEFTRIAXONE	S
CEFUROXIME	S
CEPHALOTHIN	S
CIPROFLOXACIN	S
ERYTHROMYCIN	R
GENTAMICIN	S
OXACILLIN	S
PENICILLIN	S
PIPERACILLIN	S
TETRACYCLINE	S
TOBRAMYCIN	S
TRIMETH/SULF	S
VANCOMYCIN	S

S = SUSCEPTIBLE

R = RESISTANT

I = INTERMEDIATE

M = MODERATELY SUSCEP

RADIOLOGY REPORT—PATIENT 10

DATE: 1/31/20XX

HISTORY DIAGNOSIS: Pneumonia

FINDINGS: There is slight overexpansion of the lungs. The pulmonary vasculature is normal. The heart is not enlarged. There is lower lobe infiltrate in the right lung.

IMPRESSION: Right lower lobe pneumonia

EKG REPORT — PATIENT 10

DATE: 1/31/20XX

DIAGNOSIS: Pneumonia

INTERPRETATION: EKG: NSR, widespread ST-T wave abnormalities, LV hypertrophy

LABORATORY REPORT — PATIENT 10

CHEMISTRY

DATE: 1/31/20XX

Specimen	Results	Normal Values
GLUC	281 H	70–110
CREAT	0.67	0.5–1.5
NA	142	136–146
K	4.8	3.5–5.5
CL	108	95–110
CO_2	29	24–32
CA	9.5	8.4–10.5
PHOS	3.8	2.5–4.4
MG	2.8	1.6–3.0
T BILI	1.0	0.2–1.2
D BILI	0.3	0.0–0.5
PROTEIN	6.5	6.0–8.0
ALBUMIN	5.1	5.0–5.5
AST	38	0–40
ALT	54	30–65
GGT	50	15–85
LD	180	100–190
ALK PHOS	102	50–136
URIC ACID	4.5	2.2–7.7
CHOL	89	0–200
TRIG	101	10–160

LABORATORY REPORT—PATIENT 10 (continued)

URINALYSIS—PATIENT 10

DATE: 1/31

Test	Result	Ref Range
SP GRAVITY	1.007	1.005–1.035
PH	7.0	5–7
PROT	NEG	NEG
GLUC	NEG	NEG
KETONES	NEG	NEG
BILI	NEG	NEG
BLOOD	NEG	NEG
LEU EST	NEG	NEG
NITRATES	NEG	NEG
RED SUBS	NEG	NEG

HEMATOLOGY—PATIENT 10

DATE: 1/31

Specimen	Results	Normal Values
WBC	12.8 H	4.3–11.0
RBC	5.5	4.5–5.9
HGB	13.0 L	13.5–17.5
HCT	38 L	41–52
MCV	90	80–100
MCHC	41	31–57
PLT	251	150–450

BLOOD GLUCOSE MONITORING RECORD — PATIENT 10

1/31/20XX	11:00 a.m.	310
	4:00 p.m.	300
	9:00 p.m.	290
2/1/20XX	7:00 a.m.	150
	11:00 a.m.	175
	4:00 p.m.	145
	9:00 p.m.	175
2/2/20XX	7:00 a.m.	140
	11:00 a.m.	135
	4:00 p.m.	160
	9:00 p.m.	150
2/3/20XX	7:00 a.m.	135
	11:00 a.m.	150
	4:00 p.m.	130

Enter eight diagnosis codes.

PDX

DX2

DX3

DX4

DX5

DX6

DX7

DX8

INPATIENT RECORD—PATIENT 11

DISCHARGE SUMMARY

DATE OF ADMISSION: 1/3   **DATE OF DISCHARGE:** 1/7

DISCHARGE DIAGNOSIS: Recurrent carcinoma, left lung

This is a 63-year-old female who is two years status post left upper lobe resection for adenocarcinoma. Pathology at that time revealed a positive bronchial margin of resection. She was treated with postop radiation and has done extremely well. She has remained asymptomatic with no postoperative difficulty. Follow-up serial CT scans have revealed a new lesion in the apical portion of the left lung, which on needle biopsy was positive for adenocarcinoma. She was admitted specifically for a left thoracotomy and possible pneumonectomy.

PAST MEDICAL HISTORY: Positive for tobacco abuse 2 PPD × 30 years in the past. Significant for a right parotidectomy and also significant for hypertension, degenerative joint disease of lumbar spine, and chronic pulmonary disease. The patient also suffered a stroke in the left brain with resulting hemiparesis three years ago. Medications on discharge: Tenormin 25 mg once a day, Calan SR 240 mg twice a day, Moduretic one tablet q. day and K-Dur 10 meq q. day, Proventil MDI 2 puffs PO q.i.d. p.r.n., Azacort MDI 2 puffs PO t.i.d., Vioxx 25 mg PO daily.

PHYSICAL EXAMINATION: Revealed a well-healed right parotid incision. No supraclavicular adenopathy. She has a healed left posterior lateral thoracotomy scar. Impression is that of local recurrence, status post left upper lobectomy. She is to undergo a left pneumonectomy.

OPERATIVE FINDINGS AND HOSPITAL COURSE: There was a large mass in the remaining lung, extensive mediastinal fibrosis, bronchial margin free by frozen section. Following surgery she was placed in the intensive care unit postoperatively. The chest tube was removed on postoperative day number two.

She experienced some EKG changes consistent with acute nontransmural MI. Cardiology was consulted, and she was started on nitroglycerin and IV heparin. She was eventually weaned from her oxygen therapy.

She was started on regular diet and was discharged in good condition. Her wound was clean and dry.

INSTRUCTIONS ON DISCHARGE: Discharged home with instructions to follow up with cardiology next week. Also follow up with me in the office.

HISTORY AND PHYSICAL EXAMINATION—PATIENT 11

ADMITTED: 1/3

HISTORY OF PRESENT ILLNESS: Patient is a 63-year-old right-handed female with history of recurrent adenocarcinoma of apical segment of left upper lobe of lung. She has received radiation therapy to her chest. She weighs 123 pounds. She also has chronic obstructive pulmonary disease.

REVIEW OF SYSTEMS: She can climb two flights of steps with minimal difficulties. She has a significant underbite. She has stiffness in lower spine, worse in the a.m. She has hypertension and took her Tenormin 25 mg, Calan SR 240 mg this a.m.

PAST SURGICAL HISTORY: She had a right parotidectomy seven years ago and was told they needed to use a "very small" ETT. Two years ago she underwent a left upper lobe resection at this facility. Previous medical records are being requested.

ALLERGIES: She is allergic to sulfa. Postoperatively last time she received Demerol. She also had hallucinations in the ICU for several days. She blames the hallucinations on the Demerol. The only allergy sign was hallucinations.

PHYSICAL EXAMINATION: Revealed a well-healed right parotid incision. No supraclavicular adenopathy. She has a healed left posterior lateral thoracotomy scar. Impression is that of local recurrence, status post left upper lobectomy. She is to undergo a left completion pneumonectomy, muscle flap coverage of bronchial stump. The patient has hemiparesis in the right extremities.

IMPRESSION: Recurrent carcinoma left lower lobe of lung

PLAN: Pneumonectomy of left lung. The patient is agreeable to general endotracheal anesthesia or the use of epidural narcotic. She is agreeable to postoperative ventilation if necessary.

PROGRESS NOTES—PATIENT 11

DATE	NOTE

1/3 Attending Physician: Admit for recurrent lung carcinoma, s/p radiation therapy. Consent signed for pneumonectomy. Epidural morphine usage postop explained to and discussed with the patient. She is agreeable.

Anesthesia Preop: Patient evaluated and examined. General anesthesia chosen. Patient agrees. Will provide postop epidural morphine for pain management s/p thoracotomy.

Attending Physician:

Procedure Note:

Preop Dx: Local recurrence of carcinoma of the lung

Postop Dx: Same

Procedure: Pneumonectomy with muscle flap coverage of bronchial stump

Complications: R/O Intraop MI

Anesthesia Postop: Patient in stable condition following GEA with possible intraoperative MI due to hypotension. CPK to be evaluated as available. Patient comfortable with epidural morphine. No adverse effects of anesthesia experienced.

1/4 Attending Physician: Path report confirms recurrent adenocarcinoma. Patient stable but with persistent hypotension resolving slowly—will consult cardiology. CPK MB positive. Incision clean and dry. COPD stable, arthritis stable.

Cardiology Consult: The patient has resolving intraoperative myocardial infarction. Will continue to monitor.

1/5 Attending Physician: Looks and feels well, weaning off morphine. Blood pressure stable. Left pleural space expanding and filling space. Chest tube removed, epidural cath removed.

Cardiology Consult: The patient looking and feeling better.

1/6 Attending Physician: Patient stable for discharge in a.m. Cardiology to follow.

OPERATIVE REPORT—PATIENT 11

DATE: 1/3

OPERATION: Pneumonectomy

PREOPERATIVE DIAGNOSIS: Recurrent carcinoma of left lung

POSTOPERATIVE DIAGNOSIS: Same

ANESTHESIA: General endotracheal anesthesia

OPERATIVE FINDINGS: There was a large mass in the left lower lobe.

The patient was prepped and draped in the usual fashion. Following thoracotomy the left lung was completely removed. A muscle flap coverage was used for the bronchial stump. During the procedure the patient experienced an episode of hypotension, watch for resulting MI. The patient was fluid resuscitated and sent to the recovery room in good condition.

PATHOLOGY REPORT—PATIENT 11

DATE: 1/3

SPECIMEN: Left lung, resected

CLINICAL DATA: This is a 63-year-old female with recurrent disease on CT scan.

DIAGNOSIS: Adenocarcinoma of the apical portion of the lung, bronchial margin is free of disease.

PHYSICIAN'S ORDERS—PATIENT 11

DATE	ORDER
1/3	Admit to surgical floor
	Standard orders for thoracotomy
	Tenormin 25 mg q.d.
	Calan SR 240 mg twice a day
	Moduretic one tab. q.d.
	K-Dur 10 meq q.d. in a.m.
	Vioxx 25 mg PO daily in a.m.
	Proventil (albuterol) MDI 2 puffs PO q.i.d.
	Azmacort MDI 2 puffs PO q.i.d.
	CBC
	Postop Orders:
	Admit to ICU
	Serial CPK stat
	CBC
	SMA 12
	Anesthesia:
	Morphine pump ad lib
	D5NSS 100 cc/hr
	Strict input and output documentation
1/4	Attending MD: Consult Cardiology
	Cardiology: Lasix 20 mg b.i.d. PO
	D/C IV
1/5	Transfer to floor
	Continue meds
1/6	Discharge patient in a.m.

LABORATORY REPORTS—PATIENT 11

HEMATOLOGY

DATE: 1/3

Specimen	Results	Normal Values
WBC	5.7	4.3–11.0
RBC	5.0	4.5–5.9
HGB	15.6	13.5–17.5
HCT	47	41–52
MCV	89	80–100
MCHC	42	31–57
PLT	300	150–450

HEMATOLOGY—PATIENT 11

DATE: 1/4

Specimen	Results	Normal Values
WBC	5.6	4.3–11.0
RBC	4.0 L	4.5–5.9
HGB	13.4 L	13.5–17.5
HCT	40 L	41–52
MCV	82	80–100
MCHC	33	31–57
PLT	200	150–450

LABORATORY REPORTS — PATIENT 11 (continued)

CHEMISTRY—PATIENT 11

DATE: 1/3

Specimen	Results	Normal Values
GLUC	90	70–110
BUN	27 H	8–25
CREAT	1.0	0.5–1.5
NA	138	136–146
K	4.0	3.5–5.5
CL	100	95–110
CO_2	28	24–32
CA	8.9	8.4–10.5
PHOS	2.9	2.5–4.4
MG	2.0	1.6–3.0
T BILI	1.0	0.2–1.2
D BILI	0.04	0.0–0.5
PROTEIN	7.0	6.0–8.0
ALBUMIN	5.3	5.0–5.5
AST	35	0–40
ALT	50	30–65
MB	7 H, 15 H, 12 H, 9 H	0–5.0
CPK	221, 250 H, 275 H, 230	21–232

RADIOLOGY REPORT — PATIENT 11

DATE: 1/3

CHEST X-RAY: Reveals mass in the left lower lobe. There are surgical clips in the thorax from apparent previous surgery. The thoracic organs are midline and the vasculature is normal.

IMPRESSION: Carcinoma LLL, no congestive heart failure.

RADIOLOGY REPORT — PATIENT 11

DATE: 1/4

CHEST X-RAY: Reveals absence of left lung. Other architecture is normal other than postoperative changes. The thoracic organs are midline and the vasculature is normal.

IMPRESSION: Postop changes consistent with lobectomy; no congestive heart failure.

EKG REPORT—PATIENT 11

DATE: 1/3

Normal sinus rhythm

DATE: 1/4

There are nonspecific ST changes consistent with possible evolving myocardial infarction.

DATE: 1/5

Possible acute myocardial infarction, please correlate with other clinical findings.

Enter ten diagnosis codes and one procedure code.

PDX

DX2

DX3

DX4

DX5

DX6

DX7

DX8

DX9

DX10

PP1

INPATIENT RECORD—PATIENT 12

DISCHARGE SUMMARY

DATE OF ADMISSION: 4/19   **DATE OF DISCHARGE:** 4/24

DISCHARGE DIAGNOSIS:

Acute myocardial infarction

Hyperlipidemia

Complete heart block

Upper gastrointestinal hemorrhage

Arteriosclerotic heart disease

ADMISSION HISTORY: This is a 45-year-old white male with a history of hyperlipidemia and tobacco use. He presented to the hospital with an acute myocardial infarction. He was treated with intravenous TPA and had a reperfusion. The patient continued to have chest pain with an inferior ST elevation on EKG.

COURSE IN HOSPITAL: The patient sustained an acute myocardial infarction. The patient presented with an acute myocardial infarction and underwent catheterization. The patient was found to have stenosis of the mid-right coronary artery and right distal coronary artery. The left coronary branches have minimal noncritical disease. The left ventricular ejection fraction was approximately 45% with inferior wall hypokinesis.

The patient had a successful stent PTCA to the mid-RCA with a stent. I initially attempted to dilate with a balloon, but the results were inadequate and proceeded to place a 4.0-mm J&J stent. The patient continued to have anginal symptomatology and for this reason was taken to the OR for CABG ×2. He did well after the CABG ×2 without any anginal symptoms.

The patient also had gastrointestinal bleeding following the PTCA. The patient developed retching and hematemesis and anemia for which he required blood transfusion. The probable cause of the nausea and vomiting was a reaction to anesthesia. Upper endoscopy revealed no evidence of peptic ulcer disease.

At the present time the patient has been treated with aspirin and Ticlid and has been doing very well. The plan is to discharge him home with follow-up in my office next week.

INSTRUCTIONS ON DISCHARGE: Follow up in 1 week in my office. Medications include; aspirin 1 tablet per day, Ticlid 250 mg twice per day, Tagamet 400 mg twice per day and sublingual nitroglycerin as needed for chest pain. Condition upon discharge is stable. Activity is restricted until cardiac rehabilitation.

HISTORY AND PHYSICAL EXAMINATION—PATIENT 12

ADMITTED: 4/19

Acute myocardial infarction

Complete heart block

Ventricular ectopy

Possible ASHD

REASON FOR ADMISSION: Pain in chest

HISTORY OF PRESENT ILLNESS: This is a pleasant 45-year-old male with a history of hyperlipidemia and previous tobacco use. He also has a family history of coronary artery disease. He denies any prior history of coronary artery disease, myocardial infarction, or CVAs. The patient has been essentially very healthy, except for occasional skipped heartbeat in the past for which he has never taken any medications. The patient is presently on no medications.

Two days ago, he started complaining of a dull chest ache that appeared to radiate to his left arm and lasted for a few minutes. He was brought to the emergency department and was noted to have an acute inferior myocardial infarction with complete heart block. I was consulted to evaluate the patient and proceeded with administration of TPA therapy and IV Atropine for complete heart block. At the present time the patient is in sinus rhythm and is presently receiving IV TPA. He denies any melena, hematochezia. Denies any shortness of breath, PND, orthopnea.

PAST MEDICAL HISTORY: He denies any history of hypertension or diabetes. He has a history of high cholesterol. He states that he had his cholesterol checked approximately 3 months ago and it was around 310. He used to smoke tobacco, one pack a day for 20 years. He quit smoking 6 months ago. He denies any history of coronary artery disease, myocardial infarction, or cerebrovascular accident.

He has a history of heart palpitations that he describes as skipped heartbeat in the past for which he is not taking any medications. He has never had an evaluation.

He has a history of kidney stones 2 years ago. He denies any history of peptic ulcer disease. He has a history of hemorrhoidal bleeding in the past. The last episode of bleeding was 6 or 7 months ago.

The patient denies any trauma or recent surgery.

ALLERGIES: Patient has no known drug allergies.

CHRONIC MEDICATIONS: None

SOCIAL HISTORY: He quit tobacco 6 months ago and denies alcohol abuse. He is a construction worker.

REVIEW OF SYSTEMS: Denies melena, hematochezia, hematemesis and he denies change in weight.

PHYSICAL EXAMINATION: This is a pleasant gentleman who appears slightly diaphoretic and is expressing having mild chest pain which is better from admission. He is presently receiving IV TPA. Vital signs are as follows: Blood pressure is 100/70; heart rate in the 80s. The neck shows no JVD, no carotid bruits. The lungs are clear and heart is regular rate with S4 gallop rhythm and no murmurs. The abdomen is soft and nontender. Extremities show no edema. The pulses of his femoral and dorsalis pedis are 2+ bilaterally. Neurological examination reveals an alert and oriented male ×3.

LABORATORY DATA: SMA-7, sodium 138, potassium 3.7, BUN 7, creatinine 0.9. CBC showed a white blood cell count of 12. Hematocrit 37, hemoglobin 13. Platelet count is 312. His EKG showed complete heart block with significant ST elevation in the inferior leads with reciprocal changes in the anteroseptal leads, consistent with an acute inferior wall myocardial infarction. His chest x-ray is pending.

HISTORY AND PHYSICAL EXAMINATION—PATIENT 12 (continued)

IMPRESSION AND PLAN: Acute myocardial infarction that appears to have started around 10:30 in the morning. He presented very early to the emergency department and was treated aggressively with intravenous TPA, intravenous aspirin, intravenous nitroglycerin.

We will continue the TPA and begin lidocaine. We will obtain cardiac enzymes and admit to CCU. The patient will need cardiac catheterization evaluated within 48 hours. If symptoms recur or patient does not have evidence of reperfusion will need urgent cardiac catheterization. If heart block occurs, will treat with intravenous Atropine on a p.r.n. basis. We will check a cholesterol and lipid profile in the hospital.

CONSULTATION—PATIENT 12

DATE: 4/20

CHIEF COMPLAINT: Vomiting blood

REVIEW OF SYSTEMS: This 45-year-old white male was seen in consultation because of GI bleeding. The patient was admitted one day ago with acute myocardial infarction. He was treated with TPA and later went to cardiac catheterization where he was found to have a lesion of the mid RCA and distal RCA. Today the patient exhibited hematemesis with retching. He has no past history of ulcer disease or GI bleeding.

PHYSICAL EXAMINATION: Physical examination reveals an adult male lying in bed. Blood pressure is 120/80, pulses 60. HEENT: Pale. LUNGS: Clear. HEART: Regular rate and rhythm.

ABDOMEN: Benign.

LABORATORY: WBC is 12, hemoglobin 12, and hematocrit 37

IMPRESSION: Upper GI bleeding; rule out ulcer disease

RECOMMENDATION: We will perform an upper endoscopy to be performed today after informed consent is obtained. Further recommendations are to follow.

PROGRESS NOTES—PATIENT 12

DATE	NOTE
4/19	This is a 45-year-old white male with a history of increased cholesterol, no prior coronary artery disease, MI or CVA. He presented with acute ischemia and heart block. He was given IV TPA; 1–1½ hours after TPA he had severe chest pain with elevated ST inferior leads. He was treated emergently for urgent catheter and PTCA.
	Post catheter/stent
	Procedure: Left heart catheter, coronary angio, left ventricular angiography
	Results: Normal LCA, 99% mid-RCA and 70 stenosis distal RCA, successful stent PTCA to mid-RCA with excellent results.
4/20	Cardiac: Patient continues to have pain. Will prepare for CABG when patient stable from GI perspective.
	GI: The patient experienced vomiting with flecks of blood after the cardiac catheterization. In light of apparent acute blood loss anemia will check for peptic ulcer. Probable reaction to anesthetics.
	Endoscopy Note:
	Preop: Gastrointestinal bleeding
	Postop: Gastrointestinal bleeding, etiology unknown
	Procedure: EGD
	Complications: None
4/21	Patient is scheduled for the OR today. Bleeding stable.
	OP Note:
	Preop: Critical stenosis of the mid-RCA and distal RCA
	Postop: Same
	Operation: CABG ×2
	Complications: None
4/22	Patient recovering well. No chest pain or shortness of breath. The wound looks good. Will monitor blood loss anemia. The patient declines blood transfusion.
4/23	Chest clear, no chest pain, abdomen is soft with bowel sounds. Will transfer to the floor.
4/24	Wound healing well, patient OOB ambulating, no chest pain, lungs clear.
4/25	Will discharge today. Patient to follow up in 1 week.

PHYSICIAN'S ORDERS—PATIENT 12

DATE	ORDER
4/19	Admit to CCU
	DX: Acute MI
	Cardiac enzymes q. 8 hours ×3
	CBC q. day ×3
	Meds:
	IV nitro @ 20 ug/min
	ASA 325 mg PO q. day
	Ticlid 250 mg PO b.i.d.
	Xanax 0.25 mg PO t.i.d. p.r.n.
	Restoril 30 mgs PO q. h p.r.n. for sleep
	Zantac 150 mg PO b.i.d.
	Daily PT and INR, PTT
	Diet: cardiac
	Vital signs q. 15 min ×8 then q.i.d.
	Bed rest
	O2 at 2 L/min.
	NS at 150 cc/hr for 10 hours
4/20	Lopressor 25 mg PO t.i.d.
	Social worker consult re: payment issues
	CBC at 6 p.m.
	NPO for now
	Possible endoscopy
	Postendoscopy orders
	Watch VS
	Resume previous orders
	No heparin or TPA
	Hgb and Hct q. 6 h
	NS at 125 cc/hr
	D/C ASA, Ticlid for now
	Tagamet drip per protocol
4/21	Postop CABG orders:
	Continue present ventilator settings
	Daily electrolytes and CBC
	Morphine sulfate 15 mg PO q. 4h p.r.n.
	TED stockings
	Weigh patient daily
	Routine weaning in a.m.
	Lidocaine 3 g/min
	Continue Tagamet drip

PHYSICIAN'S ORDERS — PATIENT 12 (continued)

4/22   Decrease Lidocaine to 2 g/min
        Extubate patient as soon as weaned from ventilator
        Chest tubes to low suction
        Oxygen face mask 4 L/min
        Encourage incentive spirometry

4/23   Nutrition consult re: low-fat, low-salt diet
        D/C Tagamet drip to 250 mg q. 6
        Benadryl p.r.n. for sleep
        Consult cardiac rehab

4/24   D/C oxygen
        Consult home healthcare for postsurgical monitoring

4/25   Discharge patient

OPERATIVE REPORT — PATIENT 12

DATE: 4/21

PREOPERATIVE DIAGNOSIS: Critical stenosis of mid right coronary artery and distal right coronary artery

POSTOPERATIVE DIAGNOSIS: Same

OPERATION: Coronary bypass ×2 using saphenous vein from aorta to right mid coronary artery and distal right coronary artery

ANESTHESIA: General

Under general anesthesia with arterial and pulmonary artery monitoring with sterile prep and drape, a sterile midline sternotomy was performed. The pericardium was opened. Purse-string sutures were placed in the ascending aorta and the right atrium. Extracorporeal circulation was undertaken at this point. The saphenous vein was harvested from the right leg in the usual fashion. The patient was then placed on cardiopulmonary bypass. Cardioplegia was affected. The right coronary artery was dissected. Using a 6-0 Prolene suture an end-to-side anastomosis was created between the right mid coronary artery and the aorta. A second opening for end to side anastomosis was performed from the aorta to the distal right coronary artery. Following spontaneous contraction of the heart the patient was removed from cardiopulmonary bypass. Approximating the pericardium then began closure. Hemostasis was obtained. The sternum was approximated with a parasternal wire and fascia and skin with vicryl. The patient tolerated the procedure well and was transferred to the recovery room in stable condition.

ENDOSCOPY REPORT—PATIENT 12

DATE: 4/20

Pre-gastrointestinal bleeding; rule out ulcers

Post-upper gastrointestinal bleeding; stomach and duodenum appear unremarkable

MEDS:

Demerol 50 mg IV

Versed 3 mg IV

PROCEDURE: Esophagogastroduodenoscopy

The patient was sedated and the scope inserted into the hypopharynx. There was fresh blood oozing from an area in the hiatal hernia pouch just below the gastroesophageal junction. The scope was passed farther down to visualize the remainder of the stomach and the duodenum. All areas appeared unremarkable with no other ulcers or lesions identified. The patient tolerated the procedure well. He did have some retching and vomiting after the scope was removed.

CARDIAC CATHETERIZATION SUMMARY — PATIENT 12

DATE: 4/19

PROCEDURE:

    Left heart catheterization

    Left ventricular angiography

    Coronary angiography

    Stent to mid right coronary artery

After obtaining informed consent the patient was taken to the cardiac catheterization laboratory. He was prepped and draped in the usual fashion and 2% Xylocaine was used to anesthetize the right groin. 6-French sheaths were introduced into the right femoral artery and vein and a 6-French multipurpose catheter was used for left heart catheterization, coronary angiography and left ventricular angiography. I then proceeded to perform a Stent/PTCA to the mid RCA. A HTF wire was used to cross the RCA stenosis and a 4.0-mm J&J Stent was placed in the mid right coronary artery with excellent results. The final angiogram was obtained and the guiding catheterization was removed. The sheaths were securely sutured and the patient tolerated the procedure well without complications.

FINDINGS:

1. Left heart catheterization revealed an elevated resting left ventricular end-diastolic pressure of 18 mm Hg.

2. Left ventricular angiography revealed mild to moderate inferior wall hypokinesis with overall mildly depressed left ventricular systolic function and an estimated global ejection fraction of 45%.

3. Coronary angiography (using single catheter): The left coronary artery arises normally from the left sinus of Valsalva. The left main artery, left anterior descending coronary artery and its branches, and the circumflex artery and its branches have minimal irregularities.

The right coronary artery arises normally from the right sinus of Valsalva. There is a 99% very eccentric stenosis in the large mid right coronary artery and a 70% stenosis of the distal right coronary artery.

IMPRESSION: Arteriosclerotic coronary artery disease was found. There was a successful implantation of 4.0-mm J&J stent in the mid right coronary artery. This site was predilated with a 4.0-mm balloon, then followed by the insertion of a stent.

The mid right coronary artery shows excellent results. Pending the patient's progress we may have to proceed with CABG. The patient will remain on aspirin, Coumadin, and nitrates in the hospital. He will remain on intravenous heparin while his PT levels are adjusted.

LABORATORY REPORTS—PATIENT 12

HEMATOLOGY

DATE: 4/19

Specimen	Results	Normal Values
WBC	9.3	4.3–11.0
RBC	4.4 L	4.5–5.9
HGB	12.7 L	13.5–17.5
HCT	41	41–52
MCV	89	80–100
MCHC	33.9	31–57
PLT	Adequate	150–450

HEMATOLOGY—PATIENT 12

DATE: 4/20

Specimen	Results	Normal Values
WBC	7.7	4.3–11.0
RBC	4.4 L	4.5–5.9
HGB	12.0 L	13.5–17.5
HCT	41	41–52
MCV	89.6	80–100
MCHC	33.9	31–57
PLT	Adequate	150–450

HEMATOLOGY—PATIENT 12

DATE: 4/21

Specimen	Results	Normal Values
WBC	8.0	4.3–11.0
RBC	2.88 L	4.5–5.9
HGB	8.6 L	13.5–17.5
HCT	25.8 L	41–52
MCV	89	80–100
MCHC	33.9	31–57
PLT	Adequate	150–450

LABORATORY REPORTS — PATIENT 12 (continued)

HEMATOLOGY—PATIENT 12

DATE: 4/21

Specimen	Results	Normal Values
WBC	8.0	4.3–11.0
RBC	4.5	4.5–5.9
HGB	9.0 L	13.5–17.5
HCT	26.5 L	41–52
MCV	89	80–100
MCHC	33.9	31–57
PLT	Adequate	150–450

HEMATOLOGY—PATIENT 12

DATE: 4/21

Specimen	Results	Normal Values
WBC	8.0	4.3–11.0
RBC	4.5	4.5–5.9
HGB	9.3 L	13.5–17.5
HCT	27.3 L	41–52
MCV	89	80–100
MCHC	33.9	31–57
PLT	Adequate	150–450

HEMATOLOGY—PATIENT 12

DATE: 4/22

Specimen	Results	Normal Values
WBC	7.0	4.3–11.0
RBC	2.95 L	4.5–5.9
HGB	9.0 L	13.5–17.5
HCT	26.3 L	41–52
MCV	89	80–100
MCHC	33.9	31–57
PLT	Adequate	150–450

LABORATORY REPORTS—PATIENT 12 (continued)

HEMATOLOGY—PATIENT 12

DATE: 4/23

Specimen	Results	Normal Values
WBC	6.7	4.3–11.0
RBC	2.78 L	4.5–5.9
HGB	8.4 L	13.5–17.5
HCT	24.8 L	41–52
MCV	89.2	80–100
MCHC	34	31–57
PLT	Adequate	150–450

HEMATOLOGY—PATIENT 12

DATE: 4/24

Specimen	Results	Normal Values
WBC	8.0	4.3–11.0
RBC	4.3 L	4.5–5.9
HGB	9.2 L	13.5–17.5
HCT	27.0 L	41–52
MCV	89	80–100
MCHC	33.9	31–57
PLT	Adequate	150–450

HEMATOLOGY—PATIENT 12

DATE: 4/25

Specimen	Results	Normal Values
WBC	8.0	4.3–11.0
RBC	4.5	4.5–5.9
HGB	11.1 L	13.5–17.5
HCT	32 L	41–52
MCV	89	80–100
MCHC	33.9	31–57
PLT	Adequate	150–450

LABORATORY REPORTS — PATIENT 12 (continued)

CHEMISTRY—PATIENT 12

DATE: 4/19

Specimen	Results	Normal Values
GLUC	97	70–110
BUN	12	8–25
CREAT	1.0	0.5–1.5
NA	134 L	136–146
K	4.0	3.5–5.5
CL	109	95–110
CO_2	33 H	24–32
CA	9.1	8.4–10.5
PHOS	3.0	2.5–4.4
MG	2.0	1.6–3.0
CK	1,702 H	38–120
LD	327 H	106–270
CK MB	93.7 H	0.0–3.0
Relative Index	5.5	
AST	36	0–40
ALT	44	30–65
GCT	70	15–85
LD	110	100–190
ALK PHOS	114	50–136
URIC ACID	6.0	2.2–7.7
CHOL	275 H	0–200
TRIG	140	10–160

LABORATORY REPORTS — PATIENT 12 (continued)

CHEMISTRY—PATIENT 12

DATE: 4/20

Specimen	Results	Normal Values
GLUC	97	70–110
BUN	12	8–25
CREAT	1.0	0.5–1.5
NA	134 L	136–146
K	5.6 H	3.5–5.5
CL	109	95–110
CO$_2$	33 H	24–32
CA	9.1	8.4–10.5
PHOS	3.0	2.5–4.4
MG	2.0	1.6–3.0
CK	1,277 H	26–221
LD	345 H	106–210
CK MB	68.7 H	0.0–4.4
Relative Index	5.4	
AST	36	0–40
ALT	44	30–65
GCT	70	15–85
LD	110	100–190
ALK PHOS	114	50–136
URIC ACID	6.0	2.2–7.7
CHOL	275 H	0–200
TRIG	140	10–160

LABORATORY REPORTS—PATIENT 12 (continued)

CHEMISTRY—PATIENT 12

DATE: 4/21

Specimen	Results	Normal Values
GLUC	97	70–110
BUN	12	8–25
CREAT	1.0	0.5–1.5
NA	134 L	136–146
K	5.6 H	3.5–5.5
CL	109	95–110
CO_2	33 H	24–32
CA	9.1	8.4–10.5
PHOS	3.0	2.5–4.4
MG	2.0	1.6–3.0
CK	1024 H	26–221
LD	372 H	106–210
CK MB	40.3 H	0.0–4.4
Relative Index	3.9	
AST	36	0–40
ALT	44	30–65
GCT	70	15–85
LD	110	100–190
ALK PHOS	114	50–136
URIC ACID	6.0	2.2–7.7
CHOL	275 H	0–200
TRIG	140	10–160

RADIOLOGY REPORT—PATIENT 12

DATE: 4/19

CHEST, SUPINE: There is no gross evidence of acute inflammatory disease or congestive heart failure.

IMPRESSION: No acute disease

RADIOLOGY REPORT — PATIENT 12

DATE: 4/21

DIAGNOSIS: The patient appears to have undergone sternotomy. The heart appears normal. The endotracheal tube is in place as is the Swan-Ganz catheter.

IMPRESSION: Stable postoperative chest

EKG REPORT — PATIENT 12

DATE: 4/19

IMPRESSION: Elevated ST changes. Cannot eliminate the possibility of ischemia. Complete heart block is also noted.

EKG REPORT — PATIENT 12

DATE: 4/20

IMPRESSION: Acute inferior myocardial infarction. Complete heart block has resolved.

Enter nine diagnosis codes and 11 procedure codes.

PDX

DX2

DX3

DX4

DX5

DX6

DX7

DX8

DX9

PP1

PR2

PR3

PR4

PR5

PR6

PR7

PR8

PR9

PR10

PR11

PRACTICE EXAM 2

A blank answer sheet for these multiple choice questions can be found on page 181.

Domain I *Health Information Documentation*

1. A 23-year-old female is admitted for vaginal bleeding following a miscarriage two weeks prior to this admission. She is afebrile at this time and is treated with an aspiration dilation and curettage. Products of conception are found. Which of the following should be the principal diagnosis?

   a. 634.11, Spontaneous abortion complicated by delayed or excessive hemorrhage, incomplete

   b. 639.1, Complication following abortion and ectopic and molar pregnancies, delayed or excessive hemorrhage

   c. 785.50, Shock, unspecified

   d. 998.0, Postoperative shock

2. A psychiatrist documents that a patient has wide mood swings from excessive happiness to loss of energy and crying. What condition is suspected?

   a. Bipolar disorder

   b. Major depression

   c. Anxiety

   d. Psychosis

3. A patient with a cephalic presentation anticipating a vaginal delivery failed to progress. After measurement of the fetal head and a trial of oxytocin, the patient underwent a cesarean section. What condition should the coder suspect and query the physician about?

   a. Twin pregnancy

   b. Early delivery

   c. Eclampsia

   d. Cephalopelvic disproportion

4. A 45-year-old woman underwent a carotid bypass and experienced a significant drop in blood pressure during the surgery about which documentation suggested the patient may have had a myocardial infarction. In accordance with coding guidelines, what should the coding professional do?

   a. Code complication of surgery NOS.

   b. Query the physician to determine if the patient had hypertension.

   c. Query the physician to determine if there was a complication of surgery.

   d. Code preoperative shock.

5. If a patient's discharge summary does not contain a given condition that is documented by the anesthesiologist in a preoperative evaluation and that would impact MS-DRG assignment, the coder should:

   a. Code only from the discharge diagnoses

   b. Code the diagnosis reflected on the anesthesia preoperative evaluation

   c. Code the most severe symptom

   d. Query the attending physician regarding the clinical significance of that diagnosis

6. A patient has documentation of esophageal varices. What condition may be related that may affect coding?

    a. Arthritis

    b. Liver disease

    c. Chronic obstructive pulmonary disease

    d. Erythema

7. A patient admitted with acute abdominal pain, is found to have appendicitis, and has an appendectomy. The patient has a length of stay of two days. What type of patient encounter is this?

    a. Inpatient

    b. Outpatient

    c. Long-term care

    d. Rehabilitation

8. A patient is treated in the emergency department for a swollen knee for which an aspiration of the joint was performed. The patient was then discharged home. It is important to make sure that which of the following are documented and captured for billing purposes?

    a. X-rays and other types of radiology examinations

    b. Procedures performed including the aspiration of the joint

    c. Examination and management in the emergency department

    d. All services provided including diagnostic and treatment procedures, as well as physician services

9. A patient has documentation on the discharge summary of urosepsis. The coding staff queries the attending physician about the condition and is provided further information that the patient has septicemia. This is in alignment with the laboratory tests and medication given but the diagnosis of septicemia was not documented by the physician. How should the physician be requested to document the septicemia?

    a. A brand new history and physical should be dictated to replace the one in the record.

    b. An addendum to the chart should be written.

    c. The new information should be squeezed in between lines within the progress notes of the last day.

    d. The query sheet will be sufficient to document this information.

10. The committee responsible for medical record completion reports to which medical staff committee?

    a. Chief executive officer of the facility

    b. Medical Executive Committee

    c. Discharge Planning Committee

    d. Chief nursing officer

11. Two areas of documentation in the medial record that are significant areas of focus of accrediting agencies are:

    a. Incident reports notion in the medical record and attorney's notes

    b. Past medical reports and social worker's notes

    c. Timeliness and legibility of medical documents

    d. Patient documentation and pastoral counseling

12. In teaching facilities where electronic signatures are used for residents and attending physicians:

    a. Attending's signature is all that is needed

    b. Resident's signature is all that is needed

    c. Resident should co-sign after that attending signs the documentation

    d. Attending should co-sign after the resident signs the documentation

Domain II *Diagnosis & Procedure Coding*

13. An inpatient is discharged with a diagnosis of "abdominal pain, rule out irritable bowel syndrome vs. pancreatitis." The coder would code which condition as the principal diagnosis?

    a. Abdominal pain

    b. Abdominal pain and irritable bowel syndrome

    c. Irritable bowel syndrome

    d. Observation for suspected gastrointestinal condition

14. A 55-year-old male was transferred to a nursing home for continuing care due to being placed on mechanical ventilation following complications of cardiac bypass surgery. He was readmitted three weeks later due to ventilator associated pneumonia (VAP) due to pseudomonas aeruginosa. How should this be coded?

    a. 999.9, 486, 041.7

    b. 483.8

    c. 997.31, 041.7

    d. 482.1, 997.31

15. A patient takes Coumadin as prescribed, and it is correctly administered. However, the patient develops hematuria due to the Coumadin. The correct coding assignment for this case would be:

    a. Poisoning due to Coumadin

    b. Unspecified adverse reaction to Coumadin

    c. Hematuria, poisoning due to Coumadin

    d. Hematuria, adverse reaction to Coumadin

16. A patient is admitted with lethargy, congestive heart failure, and pleural effusion. The patient underwent treatment with diuretics for the CHF, which has cleared. The pleural effusion required a thoracentesis to determine the cause. At the time of discharge, the effusion was decreased but not resolved. The correct coding assignment for this case would be:

    a. Congestive heart failure

    b. Pleural effusion

    c. Both congestive heart failure and pleural effusion

    d. Lethargy, congestive heart failure, and pleural effusion

17. A patient with human immunodeficiency virus (HIV) with methicillin susceptible pneumonia due to staphylococcus aureus was discharged from the acute-care setting. How should this be coded?

042	Human immunodeficiency virus (HIV) disease
482.40	Pneumonia due to staphylococcus, unspecified
482.41	Methicillin susceptible pneumonia due to staphylococcus aureus
482.42	Methicillin resistant pneumonia due to staphylococcus aureus
484.8	Pneumonia in other infectious diseases classified elsewhere

a. 042, 484.8

b. 042, 482.40

c. 042, 482.41

d. 042, 482.42

18. A patient has a diabetic ulcer of the right heel. How should this patient's record be coded?

250.00	Diabetes mellitus without mention of complication, type II or unspecified type, not stated as uncontrolled
250.01	Diabetes mellitus without mention of complication, type I [juvenile type], not stated as uncontrolled
250.02	Diabetes mellitus without mention of complication, type II or unspecified type, uncontrolled
250.03	Diabetes mellitus without mention of complication, type I [juvenile type], uncontrolled
250.60	Diabetes with neurological manifestations, type II or unspecified type, not stated as uncontrolled
250.61	Diabetes with neurological manifestations, type I [juvenile type], not stated as uncontrolled
250.62	Diabetes with neurological manifestations, type II or unspecified type, uncontrolled
250.63	Diabetes with neurological manifestations, type I [juvenile type], uncontrolled
250.70	Diabetes with peripheral circulatory disorders, type II or unspecified type, not stated as uncontrolled
250.71	Diabetes with peripheral circulatory disorders, type I [juvenile type], not stated as uncontrolled
250.72	Diabetes with peripheral circulatory disorders, type II or unspecified type, uncontrolled
250.73	Diabetes with peripheral circulatory disorders, type I [juvenile type], uncontrolled
250.80	Diabetes with other specified manifestations, type II or unspecified type, not stated as uncontrolled
250.81	Diabetes with other specified manifestations, type I [juvenile type], not stated as uncontrolled
250.82	Diabetes with other specified manifestations, type II or unspecified type, uncontrolled
250.83	Diabetes with other specified manifestations, type I [juvenile type], uncontrolled
707.14	Ulcer of lower limbs, except pressure ulcer, ulcer of heel and midfoot

a. 250.00, 707.14

b. 250.60, 707.14

c. 250.70, 707.14

d. 250.80, 707.14

19. Assign code(s) for the following diagnosis: Congestive heart failure due to hypertension.

401.9	Essential hypertension, unspecified
402.90	Hypertensive heart disease, unspecified, without heart failure
402.91	Hypertensive heart disease, unspecified, with heart failure
428.0	Congestive heart failure, unspecified
428.1	Left heart failure
428.20	Systolic heart failure, unspecified
428.21	Systolic heart failure, acute
428.22	Systolic heart failure, chronic
428.23	Systolic heart failure, acute on chronic

a. 401.9, 428.0

b. 402.91

c. 428.23, 401.9

d. 402.91, 428.0

20. A patient has squamous cell carcinoma of the knee. What code should be assigned for this diagnosis?

171.3	Malignant neoplasm of connective and other soft tissue, lower limb, including hip
172.7	Malignant melanoma of skin of lower limb, including hip
173.70	Unspecified malignant neoplasm of skin of lower limb, including hip
173.71	Basal cell carcinoma of skin of lower limb, including hip
173.72	Squamous cell carcinoma of skin of lower limb, including hip
195.5	Malignant neoplasm of other and ill-defined sites, lower limb

a. 171.3

b. 172.7

c. 173.72

d. 195.5

21. A patient is seen for evaluation of a right orbital roof fracture. How should this be coded?

801.00	Fracture of base of skull, closed without mention of intracranial injury, unspecified state of consciousness
802.6	Fracture of face bones, orbital floor (blow-out), closed
802.8	Fracture of face bones, other facial bones, closed
803.0	Other and unqualified skull fractures, closed without mention of intracranial injury

a. 801.00

b. 802.6

c. 802.8

d. 803.0

22. A patient was seen for first- and second-degree burns of the upper thigh. How should this be coded?

945.09	Burn of lower limb(s), unspecified degree, lower limb (leg), unspecified site
945.06	Burn of lower limb(s), unspecified degree, thigh [any part]
945.16	Burn of lower limb(s), erythema [first degree], thigh [any part]
945.26	Burn of lower limb(s), blisters, epidermal loss [second degree], thigh [any part]

   a. 945.09

   b. 945.06

   c. 945.16, 945.26

   d. 945.26

23. Suicide attempt with overdose of Percocet. How should this be coded?

305.50	Abuse of opioid, unspecified
965.09	Poisoning by opiates and related narcotics, other
E935.2	Adverse effect in therapeutic use of other opiates and related narcotics
E950.0	Suicide and self-inflicted poisoning by analgesics, antipyretics, and antirheumatics
E980.0	Poisoning by solid or liquid substances, undetermined whether accidentally or purposefully inflicted, analgesics, antipyretics, and antirheumatics

   a. 305.50, E950.0

   b. 965.09, E950.0

   c. 305.50, E935.2

   d. 965.09, E980.0

24. Drug reaction to an antihistamine taken at home and prescribed correctly by the physician in his office. What codes should be assigned?

796.0	Nonspecific abnormal toxicological findings
995.20	Unspecified adverse effect of unspecified drug, medicinal and biological substance
963.0	Poisoning by antiallergic and antiemetic drugs
E933.0	Adverse effect of antiallergic and antiemetic drugs
E980.4	Poisoning by solid or liquid substances, undetermined whether accidentally or purposefully inflicted, analgesics, other specified drugs and medicinal substances

   a. 796.0, 963.0

   b. 796.0, E933.0

   c. 995.20, 963.0

   d. 995.20, E933.0

25. Acute peptic ulcer with perforation and hemorrhage and resulting blood loss anemia. What codes should be assigned?

	533.00	Acute peptic ulcer with hemorrhage without obstruction
	533.01	Acute peptic ulcer with hemorrhage with obstruction
	533.10	Acute peptic ulcer with perforation without obstruction
	533.11	Acute peptic ulcer with perforation with obstruction
	533.20	Acute peptic ulcer with hemorrhage and perforation without obstruction
	533.21	Acute peptic ulcer with hemorrhage and perforation with obstruction
	280.0	Iron deficiency anemia secondary to blood loss (chronic)
	285.1	Acute posthemorrhagic anemia

   a. 533.11, 285.1

   b. 533.01. 285.1

   c. 533.21, 280.0

   d. 533.20, 280.0

26. Assign the *best* answer to complete the following sentence. The CPT codes for treatment of fractures:

   a. Use the terminology "manipulation" rather than "reduction" of fracture

   b. Include internal fixation in all codes

   c. Do not include application of cast

   d. Do not differentiate between open and closed treatment; CPT only specifies the site of the fracture

27. In CPT, if a patient has two lacerations of the arm that are repaired with simple closures, the coder would assign:

   a. Two CPT codes expressing each laceration repair

   b. One CPT code for the largest laceration

   c. One CPT code, adding the lengths of the lacerations together

   d. One CPT code for the most complex closure

28. According to CPT, a repair of a laceration that includes retention sutures would be considered what type of closure?

   a. Simple

   b. Intermediate

   c. Not specified

   d. Complex

29. The patient was monitored under general anesthesia for keratoplasty including excision of diseased cornea. A controlled depth-setting blade was used to cut partially into the recipient's cornea in a manner to allow the lamellar graft to fit. Which CPT code should be assigned?

65710	Keratoplasty (corneal transplant); anterior lamellar
65730	Keratoplasty (corneal transplant); penetrating (except in aphakia or pseudophakia)
65750	Keratoplasty (corneal transplant); penetrating (in aphakia)
65755	Keratoplasty (corneal transplant); penetrating (in pseudophakia)

   a. 65710

   b. 65730

   c. 65750

   d. 65755

30. Assign the correct CPT code for a 50-year-old female patient admitted to outpatient surgery department for laparoscopic surgical repair of a recurrent, incarcerated incisional hernia with mesh insertion.

49561	Repair initial incisional or ventral hernia; incarcerated or strangulated
49566	Repair recurrent incisional or ventral hernia; incarcerated or strangulated
49657	Laparoscopy, surgical, repair, recurrent incisional hernia (includes mesh insertion, when performed); incarcerated or strangulated
49565	Repair recurrent incisional or ventral hernia, reducible

   a. 49561

   b. 49566

   c. 49657

   d. 49565

31. Patient with renal tumors received percutaneous cryotherapy ablation of three tumors on the right kidney in the same operative episode at Memorial Hospital. Assign a CPT code for this procedure.

50592	Ablation, 1 or more renal tumor(s), percutaneous, unilateral, radiofrequency
50593	Ablation, renal tumor(s), unilateral, percutaneous, cryotherapy
50590	Lithotripsy, extracorporeal shock wave
50250	Ablation, open, 1 or more renal mass lesion(s), cryosurgical, including intraoperative ultrasound guidance and monitoring, if performed

   a. 50592

   b. 50593

   c. 50590

   d. 50250

32. In outpatient surgery, a PTCA is completed with insertion of a drug-eluting stent in the left circumflex artery and a non-drug-eluting stent inserted into the left anterior descending artery of this 56-year-old female. Assign the correct CPT code(s) for this procedure.

92920	Percutaneous transluminal coronary angioplasty; single major coronary artery or branch
+92921	each additional branch of a major coronary artery (List separately in additional to code for primary procedure)
92928	Percutaneous transcatheter placement of intracoronary stent(s), with coronary angioplasty when performed; single major coronary artery or branch
+92929	each additional branch of a major coronary artery (List separately in addition to code for primary procedure)
G0290	Transcatheter placement of a drug eluting intracoronary stent(s), percutaneous, with or without other therapeutic intervention, any method; single vessel
G0291	Transcatheter placement of a drug eluting intracoronary stent(s), percutaneous, with or without other therapeutic intervention, any method; each additional vessel
–LC	Left circumflex coronary artery
–LD	Left anterior descending coronary artery

a. 92921, 92920

b. 92920, 92921

c. G0291–LC

d. G0290–LC

33. Patient admitted for laparoscopic repair of diaphragmatic hernia via abdominal approach. Assign the ICD-9-CM procedure code for this surgery.

53.71	Laparoscopic repair of diaphragmatic hernia, abdominal approach
53.72	Other and open repair of diaphragmatic hernia, abdominal approach
53.83	Laparoscopic repair of diaphragmatic hernia, with thoracic approach
53.84	Other and open repair of diaphragmatic hernia, with thoracic approach

a. 53.71

b. 53.72

c. 53.83

d. 53.84

34. Patient presents in the ER with thrombosis of a loop PTFE hemodialysis fistula without mechanical complications. The physician performed a thrombectomy of the left forearm graft. Assign a facility code for this outpatient procedure.

39.49	Other revision of vascular procedure
36831	Thrombectomy, open, arteriovenous fistula without revision, autogenous or nonautogenous dialysis graft (separate procedure)
36832	Revision, open, arteriovenous fistula; without thrombectomy, autogenous or nonautogenous dialysis graft (separate procedure)
37184	Primary percutaneous transluminal mechanical thrombectomy, noncoronary, arterial or arterial bypass graft, including fluoroscopic guidance and intraprocedural pharmacological thrombolytic injection(s); initial vessel

a. 39.49

b. 36831

c. 37184

d. 36832

35. Physician performed a myringotomy under general anesthesia for insertion of ventilating tubes bilaterally on a 4-year-old male due to chronic otitis media as an outpatient procedure. What is the CPT code assignment and what modifier should be appended (if applicable) to this procedure code?

69421	Myringotomy including aspiration and/or eustachian tube inflation requiring general anesthesia
69436	Tympanostomy (requiring insertion of ventilating tube), general anesthesia
–50	Bilateral procedure
–51	Multiple procedures
–RT	Right side
–LT	Left side

a. 69421–RT

b. 69421–LT

c. 69436–51

d. 69436–50

36. Removal of two (2) skin tags on chest (0.3 cm and 0.5 cm). What is the correct CPT code(s) assignment?

11200	Removal of skin tags, multiple fibrocutaneous tags, any area; up to and including 15 lesions
11201	Removal of skin tags, multiple fibrocutaneous tags, any area; each additional 10 lesions, or part thereof (List separately in additional to code for primary procedure.)
11305	Shaving of epidermal or dermal lesion, single lesion, scalp neck, hands, feet, genitalia; lesion diameter 0.5 cm or less

a. 11200, 11201

b. 11305, 11305

c. 11305

d. 11200

37. In outpatient surgery, a patient undergoes a direct laryngoscopy with operating microscope. What code should be assigned?

31515	Laryngoscopy direct, with or without tracheoscopy; for aspiration
31520	Laryngoscopy direct, with or without tracheoscopy; diagnostic newborn
31525	Laryngoscopy direct, with or without tracheoscopy; diagnostic except newborn
31526	Laryngoscopy direct, with or without tracheoscopy; diagnostic, with operating microscope or telescope

    a. 31515

    b. 31520

    c. 31525

    d. 31526

Domain III   *Regulatory Guidelines and Reporting Requirements for Acute-Care (Inpatient) Service*

38. According to the UHDDS, the definition of a *secondary diagnosis* is a condition that:

    a. Is recorded in the patient record

    b. Receives evaluation and is documented by the physician

    c. Receives clinical evaluation, therapeutic treatment, further evaluation, extends the length of stay, increases nursing monitoring and care

    d. Is considered to be essential by the physicians involved and is reflected in the record

39. A female patient is diagnosed with congestive heart failure and also has a stage IV pressure ulcer. Which of the following indicators must be present so that the ulcer will be classified as a MCC for this admission?

    a. N

    b. Y

    c. W

    d. U

40. A patient is admitted to a healthcare facility with ataxia and syncope. The patient has a history of lung cancer. The patient also has a fractured arm as a result of falling. The patient undergoes a closed reduction of the fracture in the emergency department and a complete workup for metastatic carcinoma of the brain. The patient is found to have metastatic carcinoma of the lung to the brain and undergoes radiation therapy to the brain. The principal diagnosis should be:

    a. Fractured arm

    b. Syncope

    c. Metastatic carcinoma of the brain

    d. Carcinoma of the lung

41. A 78-year-old patient is admitted with shortness of breath and a chest x-ray reveals infiltrates in the lung with pleural effusion. The patient also has a history of hypertension with left ventricular hypertrophy. The patient is given Lasix and the shortness of breath is relieved. From the information given, what is the probable principal diagnosis?

   a. Pneumonia

   b. Congestive heart failure

   c. Pleural effusion

   d. Chronic obstructive pulmonary disease

42. A patient is admitted with abdominal pain. The discharge documentation specifies "pancreatitis vs. noncalculus cholecystitis" as the final diagnoses. Both diagnoses are equally treated. Based on coding guidelines, the correct conditions that could be assigned codes and the sequencing for them in this case would be:

   a. Sequence either the pancreatitis or noncalculus cholecystitis first

   b. Pancreatitis; noncalculus cholecystitis; abdominal pain

   c. Noncalculus cholecystitis; pancreatitis

   d. Sequence the abdominal pain first, followed by pancreatitis and noncalculus cholecystitis as secondary diagnoses

43. An inpatient undergoes a procedure and has a postoperative complication during the hospitalization. The insurance company will not pay for the entire amount requested. Which POA indicator is likely part of the cause?

   a. N

   b. Y

   c. W

   d. U

44. The best answer to describe how the UHDDS defines a comorbidity is a diagnosis that:

   a. Affects the payment rate

   b. Occurs after admission

   c. Is not documented

   d. Pre-exists before admission

45. A significant procedure is one that requires all of the following *except*:

   a. Is surgical in nature

   b. Carries a genetic risk

   c. Carries an anesthetic risk

   d. Requires specialized training

46. The Uniform Bill-2004 supports, among other things, the transition to:

   a. An integrated health care delivery system

   b. A morbidity registry system

   c. Increased patient empowerment

   d. ICD-10-CM and ICD-10-PCS

47. A condition that is established after study to be chiefly responsible for the admission is the:

    a. Reason for visit

    b. Principal procedure

    c. A complication of outpatient care

    d. Principal diagnosis

Domain IV *Regulatory Guidelines and Reporting Requirements for Outpatient Services*

48. Which of the following is *not* a function of the outpatient code editor (OCE)?

    a. Editing the data on the claim for accuracy

    b. Specifying the action the FI should take when specific edits occur

    c. Assigning APCs to the claim (for hospital outpatient services)

    d. Determining payment-related conditions that require direct reference to ICD-9-CM codes

49. According to CPT guidelines, a colonoscopy includes:

    a. Examination of the rectum and sigmoid colon

    b. Examination of the entire rectum, sigmoid colon, and may include examination of a portion of the descending colon

    c. Examination of the entire colon from the rectum to the cecum

    d. Examination of the entire colon, from the rectum to the cecum, and may include the examination of the terminal ileum

50. A female patient with hematochezia presents to the hospital outpatient surgery department for a colonoscopy but the procedure was not performed due to elevated blood pressure. What is the first-listed diagnosis for this encounter?

    a. Elevated blood pressure

    b. Hematochezia

    c. Procedure not performed due to contraindication

    d. Procedure not performed for other reason

Use the information in this table to answer questions 51 through 53.

Billing Number	Status Indicator	CPT/HCPCS	APC	Reimbursement*
989323	T	10060	0006	$500
989323	T	64605	0220	$1,000
989323	X	71010	0260	$50.00
989323	S	38230	0112	$2,000

*This is not the actual status indicator, APC number, or reimbursement for the designated APC.

51. From the information provided, what would be the total reimbursement for this patient?

    a. $3,550

    b. $3,000

    c. $3,050

    d. $3,300

52. What percentage will the facility be paid for procedure code 10060?

    a. 50%

    b. 75%

    c. 0%

    d. 100%

53. If another status S procedure were performed, how much would the facility receive for the second status S procedure?

    a. 50%

    b. 75%

    c. 0%

    d. 100%

54. A Pap smear can not be interpreted because the sample was inadequate. What type of code should be assigned?

    a. Code that designates abnormal smear

    b. Code that designates satisfactory smear but lacking transformation zone

    c. Code for other abnormal Pap smear

    d. Code for unsatisfactory cytology smear

55. If a diagnosis of rule-out pneumonia with cough and malaise is specified in an emergency department visit, the coder should assign a code for:

    a. Malaise

    b. Pneumonia

    c. A cough

    d. Cough and malaise

56. Contradictory documentation may be remedied proactively by using:

    a. Communication tools

    b. External audits

    c. Compliance regulations

    d. Corporate integrity agreements

57. The National Correct Coding Initiative (NCCI) has resulted in the use of edits in:

    a. Medicare scrubbing software

    b. HIPAA software

    c. Medicare Part B claims processing software

    d. Telemedicine consultation software

Domain V *Data Quality and Management*

58. Which of the following services are paid under the outpatient prospective payment system (OPPS)?

a. Ambulance services

b. Outpatient hernia repair

c. Clinical diagnostic laboratory test performed on the same day as a surgical procedure

d. Inpatient procedures

59. What is assigned to CPT codes to indicate whether a service or procedure will be reimbursed under the OPPS?

a. Ambulatory payment classifications

b. Payment status indicators

c. Payment modifiers

d. Diagnosis-related groups

60. Diagnostic-related groups (DRGs) and ambulatory patient classifications (APCs) are dissimilar in that:

a. There is only one MS-DRG per inpatient visit with one or more APCs per outpatient visit

b. There are many MS-DRGs per inpatient visit with only one APC per outpatient visit

c. There are more possible MS-DRGs for inpatients than there are APCs for outpatients

d. There are up to three MS-DRGs per each inpatient visit while there are only up to seven APCs per outpatient visit

Refer to the following data when answering questions 61 and 62. (Note: The DRG numbers and weights are not actual numbers and weights for fiscal year 2012.)

MS-DRG	MS-DRG Wt.	Number of Patients
191	2.0	10
192	1.5	10
193	1.0	10

61. The case mix for the information provided above is:

a. 30

b. 20

c. 45

d. 15

62. The information provided shows that:

    a. The payment is lowest for patients with DRG 193

    b. There are more patients with DRG 191

    c. The case-mix index could decrease if more patients in DRG 191 were admitted

    d. The case-mix index would increase if more patients in DRG 193 were admitted

63. Data accuracy is also referred to as:

    a. Consistency

    b. Comprehensiveness

    c. Timeliness

    d. Validity

64. A method that can be used to ensure validity of data in the database is:

    a. Encryption

    b. Edits

    c. Security

    d. Transparency

65. Data consistency means that the data is:

    a. Edited

    b. Reliable

    c. Comprehensive

    d. Relevant

Domain VI *Information and Communication Technologies*

66. The quality management director is working on physician reappointment reports and needs to focus on all physicians who attended patients with pneumonia during the last quarter. She asks the coder to get a list of all pneumonia patients who did not have an x-ray done during their stays. To perform this task efficiently, the coder should do the following: (*Note:* The same time frame applies to all reports.)

    a. Obtain a list of all patients whose principal diagnosis was pneumonia, retrieve those patient records, and look for documentation of the x-ray. Upon finding, record the patient information and attending physician.

    b. Obtain a list of all patients whose DRG was simple pneumonia and pleurisy, retrieve those patient records, and identify documentation of x-ray and physician responsible.

    c. Obtain a list of all patients who were diagnosed with pneumonia, retrieve those patient records, identify patients who did not have an x-ray done along with the physician responsible, and record this information in a spreadsheet.

    d. Obtain a list of all patients who were diagnosed with pneumonia, retrieve a list of all patients who had an x-ray from the charge master, compare both lists, and identify patients who did not have an x-ray along with the physician responsible.

67. The blood usage review committee is trying to identify physicians who have ordered blood transfusions without following the predetermined criteria during the last quarter. How can this be done most efficiently?

   a. Obtain a list of all blood transfusions given in the facility during the quarter along with the ordering physician, manually identify cases with the highest amount of packed cells received, retrieve those patient records, and determine whether the criteria were followed.

   b. Obtain a list of all blood transfusions given in the facility during the designated quarter along with the ordering physicians and lab values for RBC. Import the list into a spreadsheet and sort the data by the highest blood transfusion amount.

   c. Obtain a list of all blood transfusions given in the facility during the designated quarter along with the ordering physicians and lab values for RBC. Import the list in a spreadsheet and sort the data by the highest RBC value.

   d. Obtain a list of all blood transfusions given in the facility during the designated quarter along with the ordering physicians and lab values for RBC. Import the list into a spreadsheet and filter the data by using the RBC predetermined values or lower in the facility criteria for blood transfusions.

68. A quality improvement study showed that maternity cases are not being coded with the correct procedure code for manually assisted vaginal delivery codes associated. What HIM software could be used to evaluate this?

   a. Birth certificate registry or master patient index

   b. Transcription registry or correspondence registry

   c. Quality improvement or operative registry

   d. Billing and reimbursement abstracting system

69. The Health Information Technology for Economic and Clinical Health (HITECH) Act is providing incentives for:

   a. Electronic tumor registry software

   b. Facility-based qualitative analysis of documentation

   c. Meaningful use of certified EHR technology

   d. Revised billing scrubber software

70. The use of standard protocols to enable different computer systems to communicate is referred to as:

   a. Digital assistance

   b. A data set

   c. Interoperability

   d. Pay for communication

Domain VII **Privacy, Confidentiality, Legal, and Ethical Issues**

71. According to the AHIMA Standards of Ethical Coding, "A coder should protect the confidentiality of the health record at all times and refuse to access protected health information not required for coding-related activities." Which of the following is *not* considered a coding-related activity?

    a. Coding quality evaluation

    b. Review of records assigned each day

    c. Risk analysis of medical record documentation

    d. Completion of abstracting

72. A routine computer back-up procedure is an example of a control that ensures data loss does not occur. This type of control is:

    a. Computer

    b. Validity

    c. Responsive

    d. Preventive

73. The patient was admitted for prostate carcinoma. This was treated with radiation. A member of the medical staff who was not associated with the patient's care requests to see the patient's record. What should the coder do?

    a. Provide the record to the physician.

    b. Report the incident to hospital security.

    c. Ask the physician to come back when the supervisor gets back.

    d. Explain that providing the record would violate the privacy policy.

74. The billing department has requested that a copy of the operative report be provided when unlisted CPT codes are used. The coding staff should:

    a. Provide the report because insurers will not provide reimbursement without this documentation

    b. Not provide the report

    c. Require patient consent for this specific type of release

    d. Ignore the request

75. Confidentiality includes the responsibility to:

    a. Leave a person alone

    b. Limit disclosure of private matters

    c. Provide physical protection of information

    d. Disclose anything requested

76. In most circumstances, the person who authorizes release of medical information is:

    a. Chief executive officer

    b. Patient

    c. Physician

    d. Nurse

Domain VIII *Compliance*

77. According to Medicare requirements, a history and physical must:

    a. Be coded based on the uniform hospital discharge proposal

    b. Include the patient's weight, height, body mass index, and year of birth

    c. Be completed for each patient no more than 30 days before or 24 hours after admission or registration, but prior to surgery

    d. Discuss the educational plans for the patient including diet, exercise, and plans for smoking cessation

78. Which of the following is a key part of an internal coding compliance plan for facility-based evaluation and management code assignment?

    a. Regular internal audits comparing the code assignment to the facility guidelines

    b. Audits performed by objective external reviewers

    c. Coding audits performed by physician payers

    d. Sharing and discussing results with admission staff

79. Proper discharge planning for inpatients being transferred to another healthcare delivery system must include a complete summary of the patient's history, current status, and future needs to ensure appropriate:

    a. Coding

    b. Billing

    c. Continuity of care

    d. Quality of care

80. Which of the following is *not* part of a coding compliance plan?

    a. Regular internal audits

    b. Audits performed by objective external reviewers

    c. Coding audits performed by payers

    d. Sharing and discussing results with coding staff

81. Based on the "Compliance Program Guidance for Hospitals," identify which of the following is *not* one of the seven elements specified by the Office of the Inspector General (OIG):

    a. Written standards of conduct

    b. Development of a penalty fund

    c. Designation of a Chief Compliance Officer

    d. A system to respond to allegations

Multiple Select Questions

Please select all answers that apply for the following multiple select questions:

82. If a patient is admitted with a substance-related psychosis, what is coded? (Select all that apply.)

    a. The psychosis is coded first.

    b. The drug or alcohol dependence is coded first.

    c. The drug or alcohol dependence is coded second.

    d. The psychosis is not coded.

    e. The drug or alcohol dependence is not coded.

    f. Only a history of drug or alcohol dependence is coded.

83. When coding a documented ventilator associated pneumonia (VAP) what codes should be assigned? (Select all that apply.)

    a. The pneumonia is coded first.

    b. The complication of surgery is coded first.

    c. The specific code for ventilator associated pneumonia is coded first.

    d. An additional code for the type of pneumonia, that is, lobar or pneumonia NOS, is not coded.

    e. The organism is coded as a secondary code if known.

    f. An additional code for the type of pneumonia, that is, lobar or pneumonia NOS, is coded.

84. When trying to determine if documentation is present to substantiate status asthmaticus the coder should review the record for what terms and phrases? (Select all that apply.)

    a. Intractable pneumonia

    b. Refractory asthma

    c. Severe, intractable wheezing

    d. Airway obstruction not relieved by bronchodilators

    e. Limited but pronounced wheezing

    f. Severe, prolonged asthma attack

85. Gastrointestinal bleeding manifests itself in several ways. (Select all that apply.)

    a. Hematemesis which indicates acute upper gastrointestinal hemorrhage

    b. Petechia

    c. Melena which indicates upper or lower gastrointestinal hemorrhage

    d. Constipation which indicates upper or lower gastrointestinal hemorrhage

    e. Occult bleeding which indicates upper or lower gastrointestinal hemorrhage

    f. Hematochezia which indicates lower gastrointestinal hemorrhage

86. Mechanical ventilation codes require consideration of which of the following? (Select all that apply.)

    a. The time when a tracheal tube is inserted

    b. The replacement of an endotracheal tube

    c. The start time of endotracheal tube insertion followed by mechanical ventilation

    d. Mechanical ventilation during surgery

    e. Time that a patient on mechanical ventilation is admitted

    f. Discontinuance of mechanical ventilation

87. Examples of breast reconstruction include which of the following? (Select all that apply.)

    a. Total reconstruction

    b. Insertion of drains

    c. Flaps and microsurgical procedures

    d. Nipple-areola reconstruction

    e. Removal of lymph nodes

    f. Reduction mammoplasty

88. Name the three types of pacemaker devices that each have a unique ICD-9-CM code. (Select all that apply.)

    a. Dual chamber rate responsive

    b. Single chamber

    c. Multiple chamber

    d. Single chamber rate responsive

    e. Multiple chamber rate responsive

    f. Dual chamber

89. If a patient undergoes a biopsy immediately before the definitive surgery for a frozen section, how should this be coded with ICD-9-CM codes? (Select all that apply.)

    a. The approach to the definitive surgery

    b. Suture method

    c. Exploratory surgery

    d. Open biopsy

    e. Definitive surgery

    f. Closure of the operative site

Multiple Choice and Multiple Select Exam 2 Answers

1.	24.	47.	70.
2.	25.	48.	71.
3.	26.	49.	72.
4.	27.	50.	73.
5.	28.	51.	74.
6.	29.	52.	75.
7.	30.	53.	76.
8.	31.	54.	77.
9.	32.	55.	78.
10.	33.	56.	79.
11.	34.	57.	80.
12.	35.	58.	81.
13.	36.	59.	82.
14.	37.	60.	83.
15.	38.	61.	84.
16.	39.	62.	85.
17.	40.	63.	86.
18.	41.	64.	87.
19.	42.	65.	88.
20.	43.	66.	89.
21.	44.	67.	
22.	45.	68.	
23.	46.	69.	

PRACTICE EXAM 2
CASE STUDIES

*Note: Review the Procedures for Coding Medical Record Cases
for the CCS Examination in the Introduction of this book.*

SAME-DAY SURGERY RECORD—PATIENT 1

DATE OF ADMISSION: 1/29   **DATE OF DISCHARGE:** 1/29

DISCHARGE DIAGNOSIS: Torn lateral meniscus of the right knee; torn anterior cruciate ligament of the right knee

ADMISSION HISTORY: The patient is a 17-year-old male, who approximately 1 year ago underwent a cruciate ligament reconstruction. He has had several reinjuries and for this reason was taken for arthroscopic evaluation and treatment.

COURSE IN HOSPITAL: The patient was taken to the OR where a resection of tear of the lateral meniscus posterior horn and reconstruction of the anterior cruciate ligament using patellar tendon graft was performed. The patient was then discharged and asked to return in 1 week.

INSTRUCTIONS ON DISCHARGE:

Levaquin 500 mg by mouth, 1 per day

Tylox 1–2 capsules as needed for pain

Follow-up appointment in 1 week

HISTORY AND PHYSICAL EXAMINATION—PATIENT 1

DATE: 1/29

HISTORY OF PRESENT ILLNESS: This is a 17-year-old male active in several sports. He then reinjured the knee several times this year while playing soccer.

PAST MEDICAL HISTORY: The patient has no other health problems.

ALLERGIES: None known

CHRONIC MEDICATIONS: None

FAMILY HISTORY: Noncontributory

PHYSICAL EXAMINATION: Reveals a well-developed, well-nourished white male in no apparent distress. HEENT reveals nothing abnormal. Chest was clear to auscultation and percussion. Heart sounds were normal with no murmurs. Examination of the abdomen reveals no masses or tenderness. Examination of the genitals was not done. Examination of the extremities reveals a scar on the left knee with swelling of the joint. Distal sensation and circulation were normal.

IMPRESSION: Torn lateral meniscus of the right knee; torn anterior cruciate ligament of the right knee.

PLAN:

1. Resection of tear of the lateral meniscus posterior horn

2. Reconstruction of the anterior cruciate ligament using patellar tendon graft

PROGRESS NOTES—PATIENT 1

DATE	NOTE
1/29	Admit to Same-Day Surgery unit
	Prep for surgery
	Betadine scrub right leg
	Demerol 100 mg IM 1 hr preop
	Versed 5 mg IM 1 hr preop
	Postop Orders:
	Demerol 75 mg. PRN pain 1 dose
	Tylox 1 to 2 PO q. 4 hr
	Levaquin 500 mg PO postop
	D/C when stable as per discharge criteria

PHYSICIAN'S ORDERS—PATIENT 1

DATE	ORDER
1/29	Patient admitted for surgical and diagnostic arthroscopy
	Brief OP Note

PREOP DX: Torn lateral meniscus of the right knee; torn anterior cruciate ligament of the right knee

POSTOP DX: Torn lateral meniscus of the right knee; torn anterior cruciate ligament of the right knee

OPERATION:

1. Resection of tear of the lateral meniscus posterior horn

2. Reconstruction of the anterior cruciate ligament using patellar tendon graft

ANES: General

Good circulation and sensation. Will encourage patient to ambulate with splint and crutches.

Discharge when stable. Follow up in one week with my office.

DISCHARGE MEDICATIONS:

1. Levaquin 500 mg by mouth, one per day

2. Tylox 1–2 capsules as needed for pain

OPERATIVE REPORT—PATIENT 1

PREOPERATIVE DIAGNOSIS: Torn lateral meniscus of the right knee; torn anterior cruciate ligament of the right knee

POSTOPERATIVE DIAGNOSIS: Torn lateral meniscus of the right knee; torn anterior cruciate ligament of the right knee

OPERATION:

1. Resection of tear of the lateral meniscus posterior horn

2. Reconstruction of the anterior cruciate ligament using patellar tendon graft

ANESTHESIA: General

CLINICAL HISTORY: This is a 17-year-old male who sustained an injury to his right knee in May during a surfing accident. He was treated conservatively before this. But because of instability and pain, he wished to have the following procedure done.

Tourniquet was used for one hour, 50 minutes

PROCEDURE DESCRIPTION: The patient was placed under general anesthesia. Airway was maintained by Dr. Spears, as the right lower limb was manipulated and found to have a positive Lachman, a positive drawer test, and a trace pivot shift. The left knee was also examined and found to have the same findings.

The knee was prepped with a gel prep, draped with the limb free. Tourniquet was applied to the thigh but not elevated to begin with. The procedure done first was a diagnostic arthroscopy, and, during this, we found that the anterior cruciate ligament was torn away from the wall lateral femoral condyle. It was quite lax as well. Attention was turned to the lateral compartment where the initial look at the lateral cartilage showed that it was fine. But on probing underneath the surface of the posterior horn, there was a partial tear but without any instability. The tear extended through the cartilage 50% to 75%. Because of this, this portion was resected back to normal cartilage, removing the torn segment. This was in an area that was not vascular.

Attention was then turned to the anterior cruciate ligament which was resected. Using a shaver, all the soft tissue was removed from around and up into the notch. A bur was used to enlarge the notch superiorly, into the lateral side and into the depth of the notch to the over-the-top position that was clearly delineated.

The first part of the arthroscopy was terminated. The tourniquet was elevated. Then an incision was made from the mid patella to the tibial tubercle, with dissection carried down to the patellar tendon. The middle third of the patellar tendon was harvested with bone graft from tibia and fibula which was sized to a 10-rom tunnel size. Two threads were placed in the femoral portion and one in the tibial portion, and the femoral portion marked at the interface between the bone and the tendon. The small saw was used to cut the bone graft from both the tibia and the patella. The patellar defect was filled with bone graft and closed. The guide for the tibial tunnel was then put in place, measuring about 55 degrees. This was placed just in front of the posterior tibial tendon and in the mid portion of the slope of the tibial spine. The guide wire was put in place, found to be satisfactory, and a 10-rom channel was reamed. The over-the-top positioning was put into placed with a guidewire. This was in the eleven o'clock for the right knee. The bulldog cannulated reamer was used, and a footprint was established. Probing revealed there to be a millimeter of bone posterior to this. This was reamed up to 30 mm in size for the graft plus 5 rom. The guidewire was removed. The eccentric guide was put into place, and a notch made. Then the two-pin passer was passed through the eccentric guide, and then the guide was removed. The exit of the two-pin passer was in a proper place on the anterolateral thigh. A guidewire was used to put in place in the two-pin passer, and the graft was passed up into the channel and seemed to fit well. A biodegradable screw was used, but the first one did not cut properly and had to be replaced after tapping the spot for the

OPERATIVE REPORT — PATIENT 1 (continued)

screw. A second biodegradable screw was put up in place. This was approximately 25 mm × 9 mm. The position and tightness were excellent, and drawer test at this point was trace, as was the Lachman. There was no impingement of the graft with extension, and no change in the length. The screw for the tibia was put into place over a guidewire, and this was an 8 × 25 tibial screw. This again was quite tight, and the Lachman test was just a trace positive.

The joint and the wound were irrigated with arthroscopic fluid, and subcutaneous tissues were closed with 2-0 Vicryl. The skin was closed with 4-0 nylon, as was each of the ports. The incision plus the ports were all injected with 0.25% Marcaine with epinephrine. The patient was given 30 mg of Toradol. Dressing was applied of Xeroform gauze, 4 × 4s, Kerlix, Ace wrap, and then the patient's brace which was a Bledsoe brace.

He tolerated the procedure well with a tourniquet time of 1 hour 50 minutes. Blood loss was nil. He will be sent home on Lortab. He will return to the office on Friday for a dressing change. He will be contacted tomorrow.

PHYSICIAN'S ORDERS — PATIENT 1

DATE	ORDER
4/1/20XX	Attending MD:
	Admit to same-day surgery
	Betadine scrub ×3 Preop
	May take own meds Lasix 20 mg now
4/1/20XX	Anesthesia Note:
	Continue NPO Demerol 50 mg IM 1½ hr Preop
	Vistaril 50 mg IM 1½ hr Preop
	Atropine 0.4 mg IM 1½ hr Preop
4/1/20XX	Attending MD:
	Vital signs q. 15 min until stable
	Regular diet
	Percocet 2.5 mg. q. 4 hrs p.r.n. for pain
	Iron supplement q.d. for anemia
	Discharge to home when stable

LABORATORY REPORTS—PATIENT 1

HEMATOLOGY

DATE: 3/31

Specimen	Results	Normal Values
WBC	7.2	4.3–11.0
RBC	4.0 L	4.5–5.9
HGB	11.0 L	13.5–17.5
HCT	38.0 L	41–52
MCV	94	80–100
MCHC	40	31–57
PLT	300	150–400

Enter two diagnosis codes and two procedure codes.

PDX

DX2

PP1

PR2

SAME-DAY SURGERY SUMMARY—PATIENT 2

DATE OF ADMISSION: 12/30   **DATE OF DISCHARGE:** 12/30

DISCHARGE DIAGNOSIS: Bunion of 1st metatarsal

ADMISSION HISTORY: This is a 45-year-old white female in good health. Her family physician has performed a history and physical that demonstrated her health is within normal limits. The patient has no known allergies, good pedal pulses. The patient has a bunion of the left 1st metatarsal.

COURSE IN HOSPITAL: The patient was admitted to same-day surgery for osteotomy of the 1st metatarsal. The patient was taken to the OR where this was accomplished. The patient tolerated the procedure well and is discharged to home in stable condition.

INSTRUCTIONS ON DISCHARGE:

Keep foot elevated.

Keep dressing dry; do not change until seen by your physician.

Use surgical shoe.

Take Percocet 2.5 mg every 4 hours as needed for pain.

HISTORY AND PHYSICAL EXAMINATION—PATIENT 2

DATE: 12/30

HISTORY OF PRESENT ILLNESS: The patient has had increased long-term pain with difficulty ambulating.

PAST MEDICAL HISTORY: The patient has no major health problems and has not undergone major surgery.

ALLERGIES: None known

CHRONIC MEDICATIONS: None

FAMILY HISTORY: Noncontributory

PHYSICAL EXAMINATION:

IMPRESSION: B.P. 130/88, pulse is 68, respirations 20, temp 97.3. HEENT, within normal limits. Heart, normal. Lungs, clear. Abdomen, soft with bowel sounds. Pelvic and rectal deferred. Extremities, normal except bunion on 1st metatarsal.

PLAN: Osteotomy with excision of 1st metatarsal eminence

PROGRESS NOTES — PATIENT 2

DATE   **NOTE**

12/30   This is a 45-year-old female admitted for ostectomy to relieve long-term pain in the left foot. The patient is good health.

D/C when stable as per discharge criteria.

Patient admitted for surgery.

OP-NOTE:

PREOP DX: Bunion of 1st metatarsal

POSTOP DX: Same

OPERATION: Osteotomy with excision of 1st metatarsal eminence

ANES: Digital

Good circulation and sensation. Will encourage patient to ambulate with splint and crutches.

Discharge when stable. Follow up in one week with my office.

DISCHARGE MEDICATIONS: None

PHYSICIAN'S ORDERS — PATIENT 2

DATE   **ORDER**

12/30   Admit to Same-Day Surgery Unit

Prep for surgery

Vistaril 50 mg PO 1 hour preop

Atropine 0.8 mg PO 1 hour preop

Postop Orders:

Continue to elevate foot.

Percocet 2.5 mg every 4 hours p.r.n. for pain.

Discharge patient when surgical shoe procured.

OPERATIVE REPORT—PATIENT 2

DATE: 12/30

PREOPERATIVE DIAGNOSIS: Bunion of the 1st left metatarsal head

POSTOPERATIVE DIAGNOSIS: Same

OPERATION: Osteotomy with partial excision of the 1st left metatarsal head

ANESTHESIA: Digital

OPERATIVE PROCEDURE: With the patient under local standby anesthesia and in the supine position she was properly prepped and draped. The tourniquet was applied about the left ankle superior to the malleoli.

A lazy "S" type incision was made on the lateral side of the 1st metatarsal head. This incision was deepened by blunt and sharp dissection until the capsule of the 1st metatarsophalangeal joint, left was reached. A linear incision measuring approximately 4 cm in length was made. Approximately 0.5 cm of bone was removed from the medial aspect of the 1st metatarsal head with oscillating saw. An osteotomy through the neck of the same bone was undertaken with an osteotome. Following alignment of bone, a wire link was placed. The joint capsule was closed with continuous suture of 2-0 chromic catgut and the subcutaneous tissue was closed with continuous suture of 4-0 chromic catgut and the skin was closed with continuous suture of 4-0 nylon.

The wound was dressed with Vaseline gauze and gentle fluff pressure dressing. The patient was discharged from the operating suite in good condition noting that vascularity had returned to all 5 toes.

PATHOLOGY REPORT—PATIENT 2

DATE: 12/30

SPECIMEN: Bunion from the 1st toe left foot

GROSS DESCRIPTION: The specimen consists of a dome-shaped fragment of hypertrophic osseous tissue that measures $1.2 \times 1.1 \times 0.5$ cm. Decalcification.

MICROSCOPIC DESCRIPTION: Sections of the decalcified tissue reveal fragments of hypertrophic osteocartilaginous tissue. No evidence of metastatic disease or neutrophilic inflammatory infiltrate was noted.

DIAGNOSIS: Bone (left 1st toe): Fragments of hypertrophic osteocartilaginous tissue

Enter one diagnosis code and one procedure code.

PDX

PP1

Emergency Department Evaluation and Management (E/M) Mapping Scenario for Emergency Department Cases 3 and 4

Code the procedures that are done in the emergency department as well as the E/M code derived from the E/M mapping scenario.

Point Value Key

Level 1 = 1–20

Level 2 = 21–35

Level 3 = 36–47

Level 4 = 48–60

Level 5 = > 61

Critical Care > 61 with constant physician attendance

CPT Codes

Level 1   99281   99281–25 with procedure/laboratory/radiology

Level 2   99282   99282–25 with procedure/laboratory/radiology

Level 3   99283   99283–25 with procedure/laboratory/radiology

Level 4   99284   99284–25 with procedure/laboratory/radiology

Level 5   99285   99285–25 with procedure/laboratory/radiology

Emergency Department Acuity Points					
	5	10	15	20	25
Meds Given	1–2	3–5	6–7	8–9	> 10
Extent of Hx	Brief	PF	EPF	Detail	Comprehensive
Extent of Examination	Brief	PF	EPF	Detail	Comprehensive
Number of Tests Ordered	0–1	2–3	4–5	6–7	> 8
Supplies Used	1	2–3	4–5	6–7	> 8

EMERGENCY DEPARTMENT RECORD—PATIENT 3

DATE OF ADMISSION: 8/19   **DATE OF DISCHARGE:** 8/19

HISTORY (Problem Focused):

ADMISSION HISTORY: This is a 13-year-old African-American male. He became short of breath, used his inhaler as described but continued to have wheezing and shortness of breath.

ALLERGIES: None

CHRONIC MEDICATIONS: Albuterol inhaler

FAMILY HISTORY: Noncontributory

SOCIAL HISTORY: The patient's father smokes one pack of cigarettes per day but he does not smoke in the house.

REVIEW OF SYSTEMS: His integumentary, musculoskeletal, cardiovascular, genitourinary, and gastrointestinal systems are negative.

PHYSICAL EXAMINATION (Extended Problem Focused):

GENERAL APPEARANCE: This is an alert, cooperative young male in acute distress.

HEENT: PERRLA, extraocular movements are full

NECK: Supple

CHEST: Lungs reveal wheezes and rales. Heart has normal sinus rhythm.

ABDOMEN: Soft and nontender, no organomegaly

EXTREMITIES: Examination is normal.

LABORATORY DATA: Urinalysis is normal, EKG normal, chest x-ray is normal. CBC and diff show no abnormalities.

IMPRESSION: Acute asthma with exacerbation

PLAN: Administer epinephrine and intravenous theophylline

TREATMENT: Following administration of epinephrine and theophylline, the patient's asthma abated. One venipuncture set and one IV set were used to administer the medication over 30 minutes.

DISCHARGE DIAGNOSIS: Asthma with exacerbation

DISCHARGE INSTRUCTIONS: The patient was instructed to take his prescribed medications as directed by his primary care physician and to return to the ER if he had any further asthma.

Enter one diagnosis code and two procedure codes.

PDX

PP1

PR2

EMERGENCY DEPARTMENT CASE—PATIENT 4

HISTORY AND PHYSICAL

CHIEF COMPLAINT: Abdominal pain and vomiting

HISTORY (Comprehensive History)

HISTORY OF PRESENT ILLNESS:

This patient was seen in our office by this examiner two days ago. At that time the patient presented with vomiting. The patient had eaten at a restaurant that night and had vomiting afterward and then some severe pain. When seen in the office, he exhibited some right upper quadrant tenderness. Arrangements were made for gallbladder ultrasound, which was performed and negative and he was given Reglan 10 mg a.c. and Zantac 150 mg b.i.d. However his mother brought him to the office this afternoon with the patient having severe abdominal pain and vomiting. He reports having had a bowel movement the day prior to examination and no particular diarrhea but severe vomiting.

PAST MEDICAL HISTORY:

ILLNESSES:

1. He had been seen last March with some asthmatic bronchitis treated with Humibid LA and Proventil MO1.

2. In December he was in with bronchitis treated with Proventil, Humibid and he was to finish Biaxin at that.

3. The patient had also seen in November of 2003, with symptoms attributable to gastroesophageal reflux disease and he was on Protonix at that time at b.i.d. and was advised to elevate the head of the bed, avoid eating before bed and avoid fatty foods plus any caffeine, cola, or chocolate.

FAMILY HISTORY: Reveals that his mother has a history of migraines and depression.

SOCIAL HISTORY: The patient is out of school for the summer during construction. He does not smoke or use alcohol.

PHYSICAL EXAMINATION (Extended Problem-Focused)

GENERAL: Reveals an anxious well-developed, well-nourished, male who is nauseated and has several episodes of vomiting during the interview.

HEENT: Not remarkable

NECK: Supple

LUNGS: Clear to auscultation and percussion

HEART: Regular rate and rhythm with no murmurs heard or thrills palpated

ABDOMEN: Soft with some epigastric and right upper quadrant tenderness. No masses are palpable. The bowel sounds are hyperactive.

EXTREMITIES: Not remarkable

IMPRESSION:

1. Abdominal pain of determined etiology

2. Anxiety secondary to #1

3. Nausea, vomiting, and dehydration

EMERGENCY DEPARTMENT CASE — PATIENT 4 (continued)

EMERGENCY DEPARTMENT COURSE AND TREATMENT: This 18-year-old male was referred from my office with abdominal pain of undetermined etiology. Treatment was initiated with IV fluids, Morphine, Reglan, and Protonix. The laboratory workup consisting of CBC, comprehensive metabolic panel, amylase and lipase and urinalysis was initiated and was remarkable only for very low-grade leukocytosis with a predominance of neutrophils and the remainder of the lab workup was normal. An imaging workup of the abdominal pain revealed mild thickening of the terminal ileum. This prompted a small bowel follow through which was notable only for reflux. The patient's symptoms improved markedly with IV fluids and the aforementioned pharmacological treatment regimen. He was discharged to home in good condition with no specific medications. He is tolerating a regular diet.

FOLLOW-UP: The patient is to follow up by calling the office for an appointment. He is to call for any recurrent abdominal pain or any other questions or concerns. Activity as tolerated.

PHYSICIAN ORDER FORM — PATIENT 4

DATE   **ORDER**

8/19

12 p.m.   Clear liquid diet
D 5½ Ns at 100
Reglain 10 mg IV q 40 prn vomiting
Protonix 40 mg po BID
CBC, U/A, CMP
Serum #5 amylase Lipase #7
Abd CT attn: pancreas and appendix today #3 #4

3:30 p.m.   Morphine sulfate 15 mg prn pain
Patient to UGI/SBFT X-ray done tomorrow
Send report of UGI/SBFT x-ray to doctor

8:45 p.m.   Discharge to home.

LABORATORY REPORT—PATIENT 4

HEMATOLOGY

DATE: 8/19

Specimen	Results	Normal Values
WBC	11.5 H	4.0–10.9
RBC	14.85	14.0–15.65
HEMOGLOBIN	14.6	12.0–16.2
HCT	41.6	37.0–42
MCV	85.8	78–102
MCHC	35.0	31.0–35.0
RDW	12.5	11.5–14.5
PLATELET	1,211	1,150–1,400
NEUT %	186.5 H	140.0–170.0
LYMPH %	118 L	115.0–140.0
MONO %	1.3 L	1.5–12
EOSIN %	0.2	0.0–7.0
BASO %	0.2	0.0–2.0

CHEMISTRY—PATIENT 4

DATE: 8/19

Specimen	Results	Normal Values
SODIUM	141	135–145
POTASSIUM	13.9	3.5–15.0
CHLORIDE	100	98–108
CARBON DIOXIDE	30.0	20.0–31.0
ANION GAP	14.0	9.0–18.0
GLUCOSE	113 H	70–110
BUN	12	7–21
CREATININE	1.0	0.5–1.4
AST	22	5–35
PROTEIN TOTAL	8.0	6.3–8.2
ALBUMIN	4.7	3.5–4.8
CALCIUM	9.1	8.9–10.4

LABORATORY REPORT — PATIENT 4 *(continued)*

CHEMISTRY–LIVER STUDIES—PATIENT 4

DATE: 8/19

Specimen	Results	Normal Values
ALT (SGPT)	19	7–56
ALK PHOS	92	38–126
BILI, Total	1.3	0.2–1.3
BILI, Direct	0.1	0.0–0.4

CHEMISTRY–PANCREATIC ENZYMES—PATIENT 4

DATE: 8/19

Specimen	Results	Normal Values
AMYLASE	85	30–110
LIPASE	12	7–60

URINALYSIS—PATIENT 4

DATE: 8/19

Specimen	Results	Normal Values
COLOR	YELLOW	
APPEARANCE	CLEAR	CLEAR
GLUCOSE	NORM	NORMAL
BILIRUBIN	NEGATIVE	NEGATIVE
KETONES	NEGATIVE	NEGATIVE
SPEC. GRAVITY	1.005	1.003–1.030
BLOOD	NEGATIVE	NEGATIVE
pH	7.0	5.0–8.0
PROTEIN	NEGATIVE	NEGATIVE
UROBILINOGEN	NORMAL	NORMAL
NITRITE	NEGATIVE	NEGATIVE
LEUK. ESTERASE	NEGATIVE	NEGATIVE

RADIOLOGY REPORT — PATIENT 4

EXAM: CT ABDOMEN

CLINICAL HISTORY: Abdominal pain

DESCRIPTION OF EXAM: CT of the abdomen and pelvis with contrast

RESULT: Helical CT was done after 150 cc Isovue-300 IV and oral contrast were given. The liver, spleen, pancreas and adrenals are normal. The kidneys, ureters and bladder are unremarkable. No aortic aneurysm or periaortic adenopathy. No masses or unusual fluid collections. The gallbladder is unremarkable. The appendix is retrocecal and is normal. There is slight thickening of the wall of the terminal ileum. The possibility of inflammatory bowel disease cannot be excluded. There is slight thickening of the wall of the urinary bladder.

IMPRESSION:

1. Slight thickening of the wall of the terminal ileum. The possibility of early, inflammatory bowel disease such as Crohn's disease cannot be excluded. If clinically indicated, small bowel series is suggested for further evaluation. Otherwise negative CT of abdomen and pelvis.

2. Normal retrocecal appendix

3. Possible mild cystitis

Enter five diagnosis codes and one procedure code.

PDX

DX2

DX3

DX4

DX5

PP1

SAME-DAY PROCEDURE—PATIENT 5

Left heart catheterization, left ventriculography, coronary angiography, drug-eluting stent to left anterior descending coronary artery

PROCEDURE: After obtaining informed consent the patient was taken to the cardiac catheterizations laboratory. He was prepped and draped in the usual fashion and 2% Xylocaine was used to anesthetize the right groin. 6-French sheaths were introduced into the right femoral artery and vein and a 6-French multipurpose catheter was used for left heart catheterizations, coronary angiography, and left ventricular angiography. I then proceeded to perform a stent/PTCA to the LAD. A HTF wire was used to cross the LAD stenosis and a 4.0-mm J&J stent was placed in the left anterior descending coronary vessel with excellent results. The final angiogram was obtained and the guiding catheterization was removed. The sheaths were securely sutured and the patient tolerated the procedure well without complications.

FINDINGS:

Left heart catheterizations revealed an elevated resting left ventricular end diastolic pressure of 18 mm Hg.

Left ventriculography: Viewed in the RAO projection with normal systolic wall motion. The end-diastolic pressure is 18 to 20 mm Hg. There is no gradient detected.

Coronary angiography (using single catheter): The right coronary vessel has dominant structure with minor luminal irregularities only. The left main is normal with the left anterior descending coronary artery having a 75% calcified proximal stenosis and the circumflex marginal system with a 10% to 20% plaquing only.

LAD stent underlying: Left anterior descending coronary vessel was easily isolated and the primary stent intervention was carried out with a 3.0 Cypher drug-eluting stent. Final sizing was 3.1 mm resulting in 0% residual stenosis and maintenance of TIMI III flow distally in the LAD system.

IMPRESSION: Critical single-vessel obstructive coronary artery disease involving the LAD system successfully treated with drug-eluting stent technology. The left anterior descending coronary artery shows excellent results. Preserved left ventricular systolic wall motion.

Enter one diagnosis code and two procedure codes.

PDX

PP1

PR2

PAIN MANAGEMENT — PATIENT 6

DATE: 1/2004

CHIEF COMPLAINT: Weakness, vomiting, sleepiness

HISTORY OF PRESENT ILLNESS:

The patient is a 55-year-old female who presents to the emergency department with her family. The patient has anal cancer with mets to the kidney-lung-brain areas. She had been seen here multiple times. She has been having increasing weakness and vomiting at home, decreased mentation. She has been bedridden for at least the last 4 weeks.

REVIEW OF SYSTEMS:

She has occasional headaches and seizures. No syncope, cough, or shortness of breath. She has had repeated bouts of nausea and vomiting, no obvious urinary frequency, urgency, or dysuria. She has had decreased mentation. The review of systems is otherwise negative.

PAST MEDICAL HISTORY:

ILLNESSES:

1. Cancer as above

2. History of hypertension

3. She has seizures secondary to brain metastases

MEDICATIONS:

Per list include

1. Dilantin 300 mg p.o. b.i.d.

2. Lantus insulin

3. Dexamethasone

4. Protonix

5. Xanax

6. Atenolol

7. Norvasc

8. Reglan

9. Benadryl

10. Antivert

11. Zyvox

12. Depakote

13. Lorazepam

PAIN MANAGEMENT—PATIENT 6 (continued)

ALLERGIES:

1. Levaquin

2. Penicillin

The patient lives at home. She is a nonsmoker. She is here with multiple family members. She is married.

PHYSICAL EXAMINATION:

VITAL SIGNS: Temperature 98.7 degrees, pulse 72, respiratory rate 16, blood pressure 142/91

GENERAL: This is an ill-appearing female with decreased mentation and speech.

HEENT: PERRLA

NECK: Supple

CHEST: Breath sounds are equal bilaterally. Clear. No wheezes, rales, or rhonchi.

CARDIOVASCULAR: No obvious murmurs, gallops or rubs.

ABDOMEN: Soft. No specific tenderness, guarding, rebound.

EXTREMITIES: Joints have full range of motion.

NEUROLOGIC: Moves all extremities well.

SKIN: Normal skin. No acute rashes or lesions.

DIAGNOSES: Pain due to metastatic anal cancer.

Upon admission to the same-day surgery unit an IV was started. She was given 500 cc normal saline. I have updated the family and written orders. I have also reviewed her records especially her previous labs as well as her history of metastatic cancer.

RADIOLOGY:

CLINICAL HISTORY: Metastatic anal cancer

DESCRIPTION OF EXAM: Ultrasound and fluoroscopic guided PICC line insertion

RESULT: The patient's left arm was prepped and draped in the usual sterile fashion. A tourniquet was applied in the axilla. The skin was infiltrated with 1% lidocaine for local anesthesia. Using real time ultrasound guidance, a 21-gauge micropuncture needle was introduced into the left brachial vein. The needle was exchanged over an 0.018 microvena guide wire for a 5 French peel-away sheath. The introducer and guidewire were removed. A 5 French dual lumen PICC line was then advanced over the microvena guidewire and positioned with the tip at the superior vena cava/right atrial junction. Each lumen was aspirated and flushed with saline. The line was heparinized. The line was secured to the patient's skin. A sterile dressing was applied. The patient tolerated the procedure well. There were no immediate complications.

IMPRESSION: Ultrasound and fluoroscopic guided PICC line insertion performed. Dual lumen 5 French PICC line inserted in the left brachial vein with the tip at the superior vena cava or right atrial junction.

Enter seven diagnosis codes and two procedure codes.

PDX

DX2

DX3

DX4

DX5

DX6

DX7

PP1

PR2

SAME-DAY SURGERY — PATIENT 7

DISCHARGE DIAGNOSIS: Severe infection on the left foot

CHIEF COMPLAINT: Infection on the left foot

HISTORY OF PRESENT ILLNESS:

This 82-year-old white female reports that she has bilateral lower extremity neuropathy of unknown etiology and she has been worked up extensively in the past by neurology and is currently being treated with Neurontin for her lower extremity discomfort. She reports that she rarely goes barefoot, but she has been in the last 2 weeks in the process of moving into a new apartment. She did walk barefoot for a time period across her new Berber carpet and noted the next morning to have sustained some blisters on the bottoms of her feet. Despite caring for them conservatively at home proceeded to become infected and she was seen in the office by Dr.'s nurse practitioner. At that time she also had a urinary tract infection and therefore she was put on p.o. Levaquin to cover both problems. She reports that her right foot improved dramatically, but the left foot continued to worsen to the point where she was unable to bear weight on it and so is admitted to the same-day surgery today.

PAST MEDICAL HISTORY:

ILLNESSES:

1. Hypertension

2. Peripheral neuropathy

3. Hypothyroidism

SURGERIES:

1. Appendectomy

2. Cholecystectomy

ALLERGIES: Sulfur

MEDICATIONS:

1. Atenolol 50 mg daily

2. Maxzide 50/75 mg 1 p.o. q.d.

3. Synthroid 25 mcg 1 p.o. q.d.

4. Quinine

5. Calcium plus vitamin D

6. Benadryl

7. Tylenol

8. Vitamin C

9. Vitamin E

10. Multivitamin

11. Percocet 2.5 mg p.r.n.

12. Neurontin 300 mg 1 p.o. t.i.d.

SAME-DAY SURGERY—PATIENT 7 (continued)

SOCIAL HISTORY:

The patient lives independently. She is currently moving into an apartment. She states that her husband is alive, but a resident of a nursing home and she is currently moving to be closer to him. She denies tobacco or alcohol use. The patient is married. She does not smoke. She is retired. She lives at home.

REVIEW OF SYSTEMS: Is as above

FAMILY HISTORY: Noncontributory

PHYSICAL EXAMINATION:

GENERAL: Reveals a well-developed, well-nourished, elderly female in no apparent distress.

VITAL SIGNS: Temperature 96.8 degrees, pulse 12, respirations 18, blood pressure 141/76, oxygen saturation 100% on room air

HEENT: Benign

NECK: Supple without lymphadenopathy

LUNGS: Clear to auscultation bilaterally

CV: Regular rate and rhythm without murmur, rub, or gallop

ABDOMEN: Soft, nontender, nondistended. Normal bowel sounds.

EXTREMITIES: Bilateral lower extremities with 1 plus pitting edema bilaterally. The right foot has evidence of previous insult the first MTP joint with minimal redness, tenderness, and peeling skin from a previous blister. The left lower extremity in the area of the 1st MTP joint is swollen. The foot is somewhat warm to touch and the patient denies pain.

DIAGNOSTIC DATA: Plain x-ray was reported as negative for bone or joint involvement though it does show the soft tissue swelling. Basic metabolic profile was within normal limits with hemoglobin 10.9. CBC showed a white count that was not elevated. X-ray of the foot showed no osteomyelitis.

ASSESSMENT AND PLAN:

1. Abscess of the foot in the area of the right 1st metatarsophalangeal (MTP) joint and the patient is admitted for incision and drainage and debridement.

2. Hypertension. Seems controlled. Will continue her home medications.

3. Hypothyroidism. Controlled. Continue home medications and check a TSH.

PROGRESS NOTES—PATIENT 7

DATE	NOTE
7/1	Podiatry: 82-year-old white female walked barefoot and got blisters on feet—eventually became infected and was seen by nurse practitioner and treated with levaquin. PE status left foot much better, but will admit for I&D and debridement. Full H&P dictated.
	Performed I&D of 1st MPJ (Left) index local anesthesia Marcaine plain 50:50 10cc. Ankle tourniquet. Less than 150 cc of blood loss.
	Findings: Ulcer deep to 1st MPJ implant. No necrosis at bone or soft tissues.
	Plan: D/C to home health to continue antibiotics.

PHYSICIAN'S ORDERS—PATIENT 7

DATE	ORDER
7/1	CBC in morning, TSH in morning
	Fe, Ferritin, TLBC in morning
	Hemoccult stool ×3
	Atenolol 50 mg
	Maxide 50/75
	Synthroid 25 mcg
	Calcium and vitamin D 600 mg
	Tylenol 325 mg
	DCN-100
	Neurontin 300 mg
	Vitamin B$_{12}$ level if folic acid level okay in morning
7/1	Continue meds taken prior to admission
	Levaquin 500 mg daily
	Discharge patient

LABORATORY REPORT—PATIENT 7

HEMATOLOGY

DATE: 7/1

Specimen	Results	Normal Values
WBC	7.1	4.1–10.9
RBC	12.90 L	14.0–15.65
HEMOGLOBIN	9.1 L	12.0–16.2
HCT	26 L	37.0–42
MCV	92.8	78–102
MCHC	33.8	31.0–35
RDW	14.6 H	11.5–14.5
PLATELET	1377	1,150–1,400
NEUT %	154.7	140.0–170.0
LYMPH %	133.9	115.0–140.0
MONO %	9.4	1.5–12.0
EOSIN %	1.2	0.0–7.0
BASO %	0.8	0.0–2.0

LABORATORY REPORT — PATIENT 7 (continued)

CHEMISTRY—PATIENT 7

DATE: 7/1

Specimen	Results	Normal Values
SODIUM	133 L	135–145
POTASSIUM	3.6	3.5–15.0
CHLORIDE	99	98–108
CARBON DIOXIDE	27.0	20.0–31.0
ANION GAP	11.0	9.0–18.0
GLUCOSE	111.1 H	70–110
BUN	18	15–21
CREATININE	1.0	0.5–1.4
CALCIUM	8.4 L	8.9–10.4

URINALYSIS—PATIENT 7

DATE: 7/1

Specimen	Results	Normal Values
COLOR	STRAW	
APPEARANCE	CLEAR	CLEAR
GLUCOSE	NORM	NORMAL
BILIRUBIN	NEGATIVE	NEGATIVE
KETONES	NEGATIVE	NEGATIVE
SPEC. GRAVITY	1.005	1.003–1.030
BLOOD	NEGATIVE	NEGATIVE
pH	7.0	5.0–8.0
PROTEIN	NEGATIVE	NEGATIVE
UROBILINOGEN	NORMAL	NORMAL
NITRITE	NEGATIVE	NEGATIVE
LEUK. ESTERASE	NEGATIVE	NEGATIVE

LABORATORY REPORT—PATIENT 7 (continued)

MICROBIOLOGY—PATIENT 7

DATE: 7/1

Specimen	Results
Feces	Occult blood negative
Left foot tissue	No aerobic or anaerobic growth after approx. 72 hours
Gram stain 07:15	No organisms seen No wbcs seen
Gram stain 20:34	Rare wbc (polys) No organisms seen
Left foot wound	Culture wound, superficial # 01 staphylococcus aureus light # 02 staphylococcus aureus light

ANTIBIOTICS—PATIENT 7

ANTIBIOTICS	MCG/ML	INTREP	MCG/ML	INTREP
CEFAZOLIN	<2	S	<2	S
CLINDAMYACIN	<0.25	S	<0.25	R
ERYTHROMYCIN	<0.5	S	>4	R
GENTAMICIN	<1	S	<1	S
LEVOFLOXACIN	<2	S	<2	S
AMOXICILLIN	<0.25	S	<0.25	S
PENICILLIN	>8	BLAC	>8	BLAC
TRIMETH/SULFA	<2/30	S	<2/30	S

S = Sensitive
R = Resistant
I = Intermediate, strains whose RiCs approach or may exceed usually attainable blood or tissue levels

RADIOLOGY REPORT—PATIENT 7

ADMITTING DIAGNOSIS: LT foot cellulitis

CLINICAL HISTORY: Severe left foot cellulitis

DESCRIPTION OF EXAM: Three views of the left foot

RESULT: Retention band wiring is seen providing internal fixation in the proximal aspect of the fifth metatarsal. The distal fifth metatarsal head has been resected, and the cortex appears slightly irregular on the lateral projection. There is an old, healed fracture of the second metatarsal diaphysis. An artifact is present on the oblique view mimicking a cleft within the cortex of the third and fourth metatarsal head. No other fracture is identified and no periosteal reaction is noted. The bones are diffusely osteopenic. The third toe appears to be surgically absent.

IMPRESSION:

1. Postsurgical change in the first metatarsal distally as described. Given slight irregularity of the cortex on the lateral view, and diffuse soft tissue swelling present, osteomyelitis cannot be excluded. radiographically and correlation with 3-phase bone scan is therefore recommended.

2. Old, healed fracture of the left second metatarsal

FINAL RADIOLOGY REPORT—PATIENT 7

ADMITTING DIAGNOSIS: Left foot cellulitis

CLINICAL HISTORY: Left foot cellulitis

RESULT: There are no prior studies for comparison. There is an area of increased density seen in the left lung abutting the cardiac silhouette laterally. This suggests atelectasis. However, would recommend a repeat view in approximately 3 months to document stability vs. resolution of this finding. There is also a large calcification seen just above the right hilum overlying the region of the trachea. There are no other areas suspicious for infiltrates. Cardiac and mediastinal silhouettes are normal. The aorta demonstrates mild tortuosity and some calcification.

IMPRESSION:

1. Probable atelectasis vs. scarring, but would recommend repeat study in three months to document stability vs. resolution of the findings in the left lower lung. See comments above.

2. I have no prior studies for comparison.

Enter five diagnosis codes and one procedure code.

PDX

DX2

DX3

DX4

DX5

PP1

INPATIENT RECORD—PATIENT 8

DISCHARGE SUMMARY

DATE OF ADMISSION: 4/24   **DATE OF DISCHARGE:** 4/27

DISCHARGE DIAGNOSIS: Stillborn infant; cephalopelvic disproportion; cesarean section

ADMISSION HISTORY: Intrauterine term pregnancy with possible fetal death in utero with cephalopelvic disproportion

COURSE IN HOSPITAL: The patient was found to have cephalopelvic disproportion and lack of established fetal heart tones for which a cesarean section was done. Unfortunately, the baby was stillborn at the time of delivery.

INSTRUCTIONS ON DISCHARGE: Continue with prenatal vitamins. Make an appointment with me in one week.

HISTORY AND PHYSICAL EXAMINATION—PATIENT 8

ADMITTED: 4/24

REASON FOR ADMISSION: Lack of fetal heart tones

HISTORY OF PRESENT ILLNESS: Patient is a 29-year-old white female primigravida whose last menstrual period was last August and whose estimated date of confinement is April 7. She had a normal, uneventful pregnancy. She was seen for the first time in September. Sizes of dates were normal with the length of time. All her prenatal visits were normal. There was no evidence of hypertension although the patient was obese and she gained approximated 30 lb during the pregnancy. No proteinuria or sugar was noted in her urine and her hemoglobin remained stable throughout the pregnancy. Initial rubella titer showed immunity to German measles. No illnesses were noted during the pregnancy that were reported or required any treatment. She was admitted this a.m. with a history of not having felt the baby move for more than 24 hours. Heart tones were attempted to be elicited by the Doppler Fetone; however, no heart tones were noted by the nurse when she listened with the regular stethoscope. She thought she faintly heard normal heart tones. No fetal movements were noted by the nurse during labor. After the patient had no progress in labor for several hours, internal fetal monitor was applied to the vertex after the cervix was dilated and the membranes were ruptured by the physician. No fetal heart tones were picked up by the internal monitor either. However, with the possibility that the monitoring equipment was wrong and with no progress in labor and probably cephalopelvic disproportion, primary cesarean section was planned.

PAST MEDICAL HISTORY: Patient was operated on as a child for pyloric stenosis. Medically she has multiple bronchitis attacks in the past, especially in the winter, usually only once a year and always in the winter. No other medical problems and no other surgeries are relevant. The blood type is B+.

ALLERGIES: None known

CHRONIC MEDICATIONS: None

PHYSICAL EXAMINATION: Well-developed, well-nourished obese white female admitted for induction of labor

HEENT: Negative

LUNGS: Clear to P & A

HEART: Regular rhythm, no murmurs

BREASTS: No masses palpable

ABDOMEN: Full-term pregnancy, LOT position. Vertex is noted to be –1 station, cervix dilated to 4 cm. No edema or phlebitis of extremities. No fetal heart tones were detected at this time.

PROGRESS NOTES — PATIENT 8

DATE	NOTE
4/24	Admit to Labor and Delivery for decreased fetal heart tones and movement. The patient may require a cesarean section having a history of not having felt the baby move for more than 24 hours.
4/24	**PREOPERATIVE DX:** Emergency cesarean section **POSTOPERATIVE DX:** Stillborn infant; cephalopelvic disproportion
4/25	Patient doing well, appropriately grieving the loss of her baby. Referral given for support group. Incision clean and dry, no erythema.
4/26	Patient is voiding well, bowels moving, no infection.
4/27	Will discharge to home.

PHYSICIAN'S ORDERS — PATIENT 8

DATE	ORDER
4/24	Admit to labor and delivery monitor Stat CBC Vaginal prep 1,000 cc lactated Ringer's solution Type and screen Prepare for possible stat cesarean section Postoperative orders: Tylenol with codeine Phosphate No. 3, 1 tablet every 4 hours p.r.n. ×4 days for pain Dermoplast spray at bedside p.r.n. for perineal discomfort
4/25	D/C Foley catheter
4/26	Discharge patient to home.

OPERATIVE REPORT — PATIENT 8

DATE: 4/24

PREOPERATIVE DIAGNOSIS: Emergency cesarean section

POSTOPERATIVE DIAGNOSIS: Stillborn infant; cephalopelvic disproportion

OPERATION: Classic cesarean section

ANESTHESIA: General

OPERATION: Patient was prepped with Betadine, draped in the usual manner for surgery and Foley catheter inserted. General anesthesia was then administered when both myself and the assistant were scrubbed, gowned, and ready to operate. Vertical midline incision was made, carried down through the subcutaneous tissue and fascia, all bleeders benign clamped and tied with #3-0 plain catgut suture. Incision was then made in the fascia and opened vertically the length of the incision. Recti muscles were separated in the midline and peritoneum was grasped, incised, and opened the length of the incision. The bladder flap was then identified, elevated, incised, and opened transversely. Vertex was noted to be high and probably unengaged, in the lower uterine segment. Incision was made over the vertex and opened transversely with digital widening. The vertex was then easily delivered through the incision. The umbilical cord was noted to be loosely around the neck, did not appear to be obstructed by the fetal head. An 8-lb, 10-oz, pale, cyanotic stillborn infant was delivered. Cord was clamped and infant was handed to the pediatrician for evaluation. No amniotic fluid was noted in the uterus in the normal sense. There was some small amount of very thick pea-soup meconium. The placenta was manually removed from a normal fundal position. Uterus immediately tightened up. Pitocin was added to the intravenous line. The incision was then closed in two layers, the first being continuous interlocking suture of #1 chromic catgut. No bleeding was noted from the incision. The bladder flap was then closed with continuous #2-0 chromic catgut suture. All blood was removed from the pelvis. Incision was clean and no bleeding was noted. Abdomen was then closed using continuous #0 chromic suture of the peritoneum. Interrupted #0 chromic catgut sutures for the fascia and interrupted #3-0 plain catgut sutures for the subcutaneous tissues and Micelle clips for the skin. Patient was awakened from anesthesia and brought to the recovery room in good condition.

LABORATORY REPORTS — PATIENT 8

HEMATOLOGY

DATE: 4/24

Specimen	Results	Normal Values
WBC	5.0	4.3–11.0
RBC	4.7	4.5–5.9
HGB	13.6	13.5–17.5
HCT	42	41–52
MCV	90	80–100
MCHC	40	31–57
PLT	250	150–450

Enter six diagnosis codes and three procedure codes.

PDX

DX2

DX3

DX4

DX5

DX6

PP1

PR2

PR3

INPATIENT RECORD—PATIENT 9

DISCHARGE SUMMARY

DATE OF ADMISSION: 9/25   **DATE OF DISCHARGE:** 9/26

DISCHARGE DIAGNOSIS:

1. Diarrhea and Dehydration due to overdose of Sinemet

2. Parkinson's disease

3. Hypertension

4. Stage V chronic kidney disease

5. CHF

Patient is a 75-year-old woman with a history of severe Parkinson's disease admitted on 9/25 and discharged with a diagnosis of diarrhea and dehydration.

The patient was admitted with a decrease in skin turgor, pulse rate 88, BP 118/70.

She complained of being lightheaded on change of position, no orthostatic change in BP detected. Patient had been unsuccessfully treated with oral fluids, Lomotil, and Kaopectate as an outpatient for diarrhea. Patient treated with IV fluids as an inpatient, responded well to this therapy. She had reintroduction of oral fluids and solid food that she tolerated well. The etiology of her GI complaints were thought to be due to an overdose of Sinemet. Throat cultures for pathogen and bacteria were negative. CBC showed WBC 9,200 with normal differential. Hct 38.1, SMA-6 consistent with mild dehydration and CRF. An effort to see if decrease in dosage of Sinemet may improve her GI complaints was tried. We decreased her Sinemet to 3 times per day, dosage of 25 100-mg tablets.

Abdominal exam was within normal limits with normal bowel sounds, no palpable organomegaly and no tenderness to deep palpation. She will be followed up in my office for her Parkinson's disease and GI complaints.

HISTORY AND PHYSICAL EXAMINATION—PATIENT 9

ADMITTED: 9/25

REASON FOR ADMISSION: Dehydration, diarrhea due to overdose of Sinemet, Parkinson's disease

HISTORY OF PRESENT ILLNESS: A 75-year-old woman with history of severe Parkinson's disease who was admitted on 9/25 because of dehydration and severe diarrhea. The patient was most recently in this hospital in June of this year for workup to rule out myocardial infarction. Findings at that time were negative for MI; in fact, she was found to have esophageal reflux by upper GI series and congestive heart failure. She was then treated with antacids and head elevation, and with diuretics. She accidently took two doses of Sinemet each day. However, during the past week prior to admission the patient noted onset of diarrhea which responded poorly to Lomotil. She continued to take two doses of Sinemet as well as Kaopectate and Lomotil p.r.n. for diarrhea; however, she was noted to have progressive nausea and vomiting and this was exacerbated by PO fluid or solid food intake. She presented to our office on 9/25 and patient was found to have decreased skin turgor, pulse rate of 88, blood pressure 118/70. The patient complained of being lightheaded on change of position. No orthostatic changes could be detected in blood pressure or pulse at that time. The patient appeared weak. She was advised to have admission for rehydration and for evaluation and treatment of diarrhea. Patient offered no complaints of abdominal pain. There was no evidence of heartburn. Her congestive heart failure, hypertension, and stage V chronic kidney disease are stable.

She denies alcohol use and does not smoke cigarettes.

The patient's Parkinson's disease has been fairly well controlled on Sinemet, 25 100-mg PO, q.i.d. However, the added doses contributed to patient's GI upset.

For details of patient's past history, please see old chart. In summary, patient has Parkinson's disease as described above.

ALLERGIES: None known

HISTORY AND PHYSICAL EXAMINATION — PATIENT 9

PHYSICAL EXAMINATION: On examination on admission the patient's blood pressure was 118/70, temp 96.6, pulse 90. Decreased skin turgor noted.

HEENT: Eyes appear slightly sunken. Sclera muddy. No icterus. Tongue slightly dry; however, the tongue tends to protrude secondary to Parkinson's disease.

NECK: No neck vein distention. Neck is supple.

LUNGS: Clear

HEART: No murmur or gallop audible, positive S3.

ABDOMEN: Good bowel sounds, slightly increased. There is some deep tenderness in mid epigastric area. No rebound tenderness.

EXTREMITIES: Lower extremities—no edema or cyanosis

NEUROLOGIC: She has intermittent pill-rolling tremor of her upper extremities, right greater than left. Slightly unsteady gait on ambulation. No focal neurologic deficits.

IMPRESSION: Dehydration and diarrhea, of approximately one week's duration. Of concern is overdose of Sinemet with gastrointestinal symptoms. Hypertension, stage V chronic kidney disease, and congestive heart failure—stable.

PLAN: Will decrease dosage of Sinemet to three tablets per day, hydrate the patient with IV fluids, treat the nausea p.r.n. with Tigan suppositories. Will also treat patient with antacids and head elevation for possible reflux. Hold dig, diuretic and ACE for now. Hold Calan SR 120 mg PO b.i.d.

Further orders per patient's course.

PROGRESS NOTES — PATIENT 9

DATE	NOTE
9/25	Attending MD: The patient is admitted with decreased skin turgor, secondary to dehydration caused by diarrhea. Continue with PO fluids and solid food as tolerated. Hold digoxin, diuretic, and ACE for now. Hold Calan SR.
9/25	Nursing: Alert and oriented. IV running well, taking liquid diet, no diarrhea at present.
9/25	Nursing: Alert and oriented. No complaints offered at present. IV infusing as ordered.
9/25	Nursing: Patient comfortable, sleeping at this time.
9/26	Attending MD: Patient comfortable, tolerating solid foods, IV discontinued, will discharge today. Restart outpatient meds.
9/26	Nursing: Discharged via wheelchair to front door. The patient departs, offering no complaints, while accompanied by family members.

PHYSICIAN'S ORDERS—PATIENT 9

DATE	ORDER

9/25 Admission for dehydration, due to overdose of Sinemet
Clear liquids as tolerated, advance diet as tolerated
IV D5 1/2 NS at 100 cc/h
Hold Sinemet today
Tigan suppositories p.r.n. nausea
Elevate patient's head for probable esophageal reflux

9/26 Resume Sinemet 25/100 tablets t.i.d.
D/C IV
Discharge on:
Digoxin 0.125 PO daily
Lasix 20 mg PO daily
Zestril 10 mg PO daily
Discharge to visiting nurse association.

LABORATORY REPORTS—PATIENT 9

HEMATOLOGY

DATE: 9/25

Specimen	Results	Normal Values
WBC	9.6	4.3–11.0
RBC	5.0	4.5–5.9
HGB	16.0	13.5–17.5
HCT	48	41–52
MCV	80	80–100
MCHC	33	31–57
PLT	300	150–450

LABORATORY REPORTS — PATIENT 9 (continued)

CHEMISTRY—PATIENT 9

DATE: 9/25

Specimen	Results	Normal Values
GLUC	105	70–110
BUN	35 H	8–25
CREAT	1.8 H	0.5–1.5
NA	148 H	136–146
K	5.4	3.5–5.5
CL	106	95–110
CO_2	30	24–32
CA	9.0	8.4–10.5
PHOS	2.9	2.5–4.4
MG	2.5	1.6–3.0
T BILI	1.0	0.2–1.2
D BILI	0.3	0.0–0.5
PROTEIN	6.8	6.0–8.0
ALBUMIN	5.1	5.0–5.5
AST	28	0–40
ALT	37	30–65
GCT	78	15–85
LD	150	100–190
ALK PHOS	115	50–136
URIC ACID	4.2	2.2–7.7
CHOL	146	0–200
TRIG	140	10–160

URINALYSIS—PATIENT 9

DATE: 9/25

Test	Result	Ref Range
SP GRAVITY	1.015	1.005–1.035
PH	5.8	5–7
PROT	NEG	NEG
GLUC	NEG	NEG
KETONES	NEG	NEG
BILI	NEG	NEG
BLOOD	NEG	NEG
LEU EST	NEG	NEG
NITRATES	NEG	NE
RED SUBS	NEG	NEG

Enter eight diagnosis codes.

PDX

DX2

DX3

DX4

DX5

DX6

DX7

DX8

INPATIENT RECORD—PATIENT 10

DEATH DISCHARGE SUMMARY

DATE OF ADMISSION: 6/22   **DATE OF DISCHARGE:** 6/25

DISCHARGE DIAGNOSIS:

1. Idiopathic thrombocytopenic purpura

2. Chronic alcoholism

3. Type 1 diabetes mellitus

4. Arteriosclerotic coronary artery disease, status post coronary artery bypass

5. Hyperlipidemia

6. Hypertension

ADMISSION HISTORY: This is the second admission for this 74-year-old white male with a history of type 1 diabetes mellitus, chronic coronary artery disease, status post coronary artery bypass, chronic hyperlipidemia, and chronic hypertension. The patient was found to have a low platelet count 2 weeks ago. This was originally thought to be due to a drug reaction. However, a subsequent course showed it to be probably ITP. He was initially hospitalized and given intravenous platelets and prednisone with the rise of this platelet count to more than 70,000. It had been as low as 9,000. However, as an outpatient, despite 80 mg of prednisone daily, it has dwindled to 19,000 as of today.

His previous bone marrow study just showed plenty of megakaryocytes with probable peripheral destruction. There was a question of iron deficiency anemia.

COURSE IN HOSPITAL: The patient was admitted for treatment of ITP. Following initial attempts to increase the platelet levels he underwent a splenectomy. Postoperatively he experienced respiratory distress. Although platelet levels increased, his overall health deteriorated. He was pronounced dead on 6/25.

HISTORY AND PHYSICAL EXAMINATION—PATIENT 10

ADMITTED: 6/22

REASON FOR ADMISSION: Idiopathic thrombocytopenic purpura

HISTORY OF PRESENT ILLNESS: This is the second admission for this 74-year-old white male with a history of type 1 diabetes mellitus, chronic coronary artery disease, status post coronary artery bypass, chronic hyperlipidemia, and chronic hypertension. The patient refused lipid-lowering medication when offered. The LDL and HDLs are monitored via blood test each year. The patient was found to have a low platelet count 2 weeks ago. This was originally thought to be due to a drug reaction. However, a subsequent course showed it to be probably ITP. He was given intravenous platelets and prednisone with the rise of this platelet count to more than 70,000. It had been as low as 9,000. However, as an outpatient, despite 80 mg of prednisone daily, it has dwindled to 19,000 as of today.

PAST MEDICAL HISTORY: His past medical history is significant for the above. He denies recent angina spells. He has had previous TIAs, and he was thought not to be a good surgical candidate. A previous CT scan of the brain was normal.

ALLERGIES: He has no known drug allergies.

CHRONIC MEDICATIONS: Humulin 70/30 24 units b.i.d., Tenormin 25 mg PO q.d.

SOCIAL HISTORY: He stopped his previous heavy alcohol intake approximately one year ago.

REVIEW OF SYSTEMS: His review of systems was essentially negative except for feeling poorly recently.

PHYSICAL EXAMINATION:

> **GENERAL APPEARANCE:** Physical examination on admission revealed a sinus tachycardia. Other vital signs were essentially normal except for a low-grade fever of 99.9. Respiratory rate was 28.

> **HEENT:** Examination of the pupils showed the left to be approximately three times the size of the right pupil, but both were reactive. There was normal extraocular movement.

> **NECK:** There was no jugular venous distention.

> **LUNGS:** Clear to auscultation and percussion.

> **HEART:** Cardiac examination revealed a loud S1 and sinus tachycardia.

> **ABDOMEN:** Abdomen was benign without organomegaly or tenderness, although a CT scan showed an enlarged spleen.

> **EXTREMITIES:** Extremities showed purpura without edema.

> **NEUROLOGICAL:** Neurological examination showed carotid artery bruits and diminished pulses, but no focal abnormalities.

IMPRESSION:

1. Thrombocytopenia, probably idiopathic thrombocytopenic purpura

2. Chronic hypertension

3. Type 1 diabetes mellitus

4. Status post coronary bypass surgery

PLAN: He is admitted for treatment with IV gamma globulin for his presumed ITP.

PROGRESS NOTES—PATIENT 10

DATE	NOTE
6/22	Attending Physician: The patient is admitted for evaluation and treatment of ITP. This is a 74-year-old male in stable health. He is alert and oriented. He is a former heavy drinker. Treatment with platelets and steroids.
6/23	Attending Physician: Platelet count continues to decrease. Will consult surgery for possible splenectomy.
	Surgical Consult: Patient examined. The risks and benefits of surgery explained and discussed. Patient is agreeable to surgery tomorrow morning.
6/24	Surgeon's Note:
	Preop Dx: ITP
	Postop Dx: Same plus cirrhosis of the liver due to alcohol use
	Procedure: Splenectomy
	Anes: GET
	Patient developed respiratory distress following extubation in the recovery room. Currently in ICU. Ventilator managed by anesthesia.
	Anesthesia: The patient currently in ICU developed very rapid shallow breathing postop and became combative. The patient was given Valium and he began to calm. The patient has decreased urinary output. Will increase IV to 125 cc/hr.
	Anesthesia: The patient is currently breathing on his own via endotracheal tube. Will return in p.m. to extubate the patient.
	Attending Note: The patient is now extubated and resting comfortably. Continue to monitor.
6/25	House Physician: Called to the floor to examine this 74-year-old male, postop one day. He was found unresponsive on the floor. There were no pulses or respirations. Code called, however, was unsuccessful. The patient was pronounced at 4:45 a.m.
	Attending Physician: The patient's course discussed with the patient's family. Condolences expressed.

PHYSICIAN'S ORDERS—PATIENT 10

DATE	ORDER

6/22 Attending MD:
Patient admitted for treatment of ITP
2 units of platelets
Gamma globulin
Type and cross 2 units PRBCs
Tenormin 25 mg q.d.
Prednisone 40 mg b.i.d.
Humulin 70/30 24 units b.i.d.
VS q. 3 hours
BS q. 2 hours

6/23 Attending MD:
Consult Surgery re: Splenectomy
Surgery:
NPO after 6 p.m.
FBS done before OR
Valium 20 mg in a.m.
Decrease insulin to 12 units for evening and preop dose

6/24 Surgery:
Admit to ICU
Postop respiratory distress
Vent settings as per anesthesia
½ NSS 80 cc/hr
Transfuse 2 units PRBCs
Daily FBS
Anesthesia:
Transfer patient to floor

6/25 Release body to coroner

OPERATIVE REPORT — PATIENT 10

DATE: 6/24

PREOPERATIVE DIAGNOSIS: Idiopathic thrombocytopenic purpura

POSTOPERATIVE DIAGNOSIS: Same

OPERATION: Splenectomy

ANESTHESIA: General endotracheal

OPERATIVE INDICATIONS: Uncontrolled decreasing platelets

OPERATIVE PROCEDURE: The patient was brought to the operating room where he was placed in the supine position and prepped and draped in the usual manner. Following the induction of anesthesia, an incision was made. The abdominal cavity was entered. The liver was also found to be cirrhotic. A splenectomy was performed and the patient closed.

The patient tolerated the procedure well and was sent to the recovery room in stable condition.

PATHOLOGY REPORT — PATIENT 10

DATE: 6/24

SPECIMEN: Spleen

CLINICAL DATA: 74-year-old male with ITP

DIAGNOSIS: Spleen with increased megakaryocytes indicative of ITP

LABORATORY REPORTS — PATIENT 10

HEMATOLOGY

DATE: 6/22

Specimen	Results	Normal Values
WBC	5.0	4.3–11.0
RBC	4.3 L	4.5–5.9
HGB	12.5 L	13.5–17.5
HCT	39 L	41–52
MCV	91	80–100
MCHC	47	31–57
PLT	19 L	150–450

LABORATORY REPORTS — PATIENT 10 (continued)

HEMATOLOGY—PATIENT 10

DATE: 6/23

Specimen	Results	Normal Values
WBC	5.0	4.3–11.0
RBC	4.3 L	4.5–5.9
HGB	12.5 L	13.5–17.5
HCT	39 L	41–52
MCV	91	80–100
MCHC	47	31–57
PLT	17 L	150–450

HEMATOLOGY—PATIENT 10

DATE: 6/24

Specimen	Results	Normal Values
WBC	5.0	4.3–11.0
RBC	4.0 L	4.5–5.9
HGB	11.6 L	13.5–17.5
HCT	35 L	41–52
MCV	91	80–100
MCHC	47	31–57
PLT	19 L	150–450

LABORATORY REPORTS — PATIENT 10 (continued)

CHEMISTRY—PATIENT 10

Specimen	Results			Normal Values
	6/22	6/23	6/24	
GLUC	115 H	118 H	125 H	70–110
BUN	20	18	27 H	8–25
CREAT	1.0	1.0	1.0	0.5–1.5
NA	138	140	130L	136–146
K	4.0	4.5	5.4	3.5–5.5
CL	100			95–110
CO$_2$	30			24–32
CA	9.0			8.4–10.5
PHOS	3.0			2.5–4.4
MG				1.6–3.0
T BILI				0.2–1.2
D BILI				0.0–0.5
PROTEIN				6.0–8.0
ALBUMIN				5.0–5.5
AST	65 H	64 H	65H	0–40
ALT	79 H	82 H	77H	30–65
GCT				15–85
LD				100–190
ALK PHOS				50–136
URIC ACID				2.2–7.7
CHOL				0–200
TRIG				10–160

RADIOLOGY REPORT — PATIENT 10

DATE: 6/22

DIAGNOSIS: ITP

EXAMINATION: Chest x-ray

Heart size and shape are acceptable. The lung fields are clear and the pulmonary vascular pattern is unremarkable. There is no free fluid and the trachea remains midline.

IMPRESSION: Unremarkable chest x-ray

Enter ten diagnosis codes and three procedure codes.

PDX

DX2

DX3

DX4

DX5

DX6

DX7

DX8

DX9

DX10

PP1

PR2

PR3

INPATIENT RECORD—PATIENT 11

DISCHARGE SUMMARY

DATE OF ADMISSION: 1/27   **DATE OF DISCHARGE:** 1/29

DISCHARGE DIAGNOSIS: Nonrheumatic congestive heart failure

ADMISSION HISTORY: This is a 57-year-old married white male, referred because of recurrent shortness of breath and cough. He states that he was in his usual state of good health until approximately Christmas, when he developed a persistent cough with associated dyspnea. His dyspnea was most prominent with exertion. He was treated with Ceclor at that time, with some improvement. However, his symptoms recurred and he underwent a second course of antibiotics, again with some improvement. However, his symptoms have now recurred and he is referred for further evaluation.

He has known tricuspid insufficiency, mild left ventricular dysfunction and left ventricular dilatation by echocardiogram done 6/2. He had a normal stress ECG 10/3. The patient also has hypertension.

COURSE IN HOSPITAL: The patient was referred because of recurrent shortness of breath and cough. Apparently the patient had been doing well up until Christmas. His cough was treated with antibiotics with some improvement. His symptoms, however, recurred, requiring a second course of antibiotics.

The patient was admitted with a diagnosis of congestive heart failure. He was started on diuretics with improvement in his physical examination and his symptoms. An echocardiogram was performed, which is described as above.

The patient was extremely anxious to go home and thought that the rest of his care could be accomplished as an outpatient. He is tolerating his medications and will remain on the Capoten and the Lasix and will have a follow-up appointment with his doctor in one to two weeks and I will see him again in approximately 4 weeks. It is recommended at that time that discussion for cardiac catheterization be carried out. This was discussed with the patient during his hospitalization, the reason being that perhaps his aortic insufficiency is more significant than what is appreciated on physical examination and by echocardiogram. The catheterization would aid in the evaluation of the etiology of his LV dysfunction and his left ventricular enlargement. He has also been given information about smoking cessation.

INSTRUCTIONS ON DISCHARGE:

1. Capoten 12.5 mg b.i.d.

2. Lasix 40 mg daily

3. Insulin Humulin N 14 in a.m. with 6 of regular and Humulin N 20 units in the p.m. with 12 of regular

HISTORY AND PHYSICAL EXAMINATION — PATIENT 11

ADMITTED: 1/27

REASON FOR ADMISSION: This is a 57-year-old married white male, referred because of recurrent shortness of breath and cough. He states that he was in his usual state of good health until approximately Christmas, when he developed a persistent cough with associated dyspnea. His dyspnea was most prominent with exertion. He was treated with Ceclor at that time with some improvement. However, his symptoms recurred and he underwent a second course of antibiotics, again with some improvement. However, his symptoms have now recurred and he is referred for further evaluation.

He has known moderate tricuspid valve insufficiency, mild left ventricular dysfunction and left ventricular dilatation by echocardiogram. He had a normal stress ECG on 10/3.

PAST MEDICAL HISTORY: The patient has a history of type 1 diabetes mellitus. He believes that his most recent cholesterol reading was lower than 200. He previously has been hospitalized for pericarditis and for resection of popliteal artery aneurysm. He has a history of hypertension.

ALLERGIES: None known

CHRONIC MEDICATIONS: Humulin Insulin 6 units of R and 14 units of N in the morning and 12 units of R and 20 units of N in the evening. Lotensin 20 mg PO daily.

He denies any drug allergies.

FAMILY HISTORY: Noncontributory

SOCIAL HISTORY: The patient is married and lives with his wife and smokes one to two packs of cigarettes per day.

REVIEW OF SYSTEMS: Otherwise noncontributory

HISTORY AND PHYSICAL EXAMINATION—PATIENT 11

PHYSICAL EXAMINATION: Reveals a blood pressure of 140/80, pulse 80 and regular. The patient was a pleasant, adult, white male who is in no acute distress. His carotids were without bruits. The jugular venous pulse was normal. Examination of his lungs was remarkable for fine, bibasilar rales. On auscultation of his heart, he has a regular rhythm, a soft murmur consistent with tricuspid insufficiency. Abdominal examination was unremarkable except for the presence of a liver edge just below the costal margin. He had no peripheral edema.

LABORATORY DATA: Thyroid function tests were within normal limits. Total cholesterol level was 194. His HDL and LDL are presently still pending. His blood sugar levels have been well controlled in the low 100s. His electrolytes and SMA 12 are normal as well as his complete blood count.

His EKG on admission revealed sinus rhythm with left atrial enlargement, nonspecific ST-T wave abnormality with poor R wave progression, no acute changes.

His echocardiogram revealed left ventricular enlargement, normal left atrial size at 4 cm, mild overall reduction of left ventricular contractility with diffuse hypokinesis, mild to moderate tricuspid insufficiency.

IMPRESSION:

1. Persistent shortness of breath and cough—possible nonrheumatic congestive heart failure; rule out persistent respiratory tract infection

2. Tricuspid insufficiency, left ventricular dysfunction/dilatation, by echocardiogram

3. Type 1 diabetes mellitus

4. Smoking history

CONSULTATION—PATIENT 11

DATE: 1/28

Podiatric consultation was requested. The patient's chart was reviewed in the following manner:

H & P, Labs, progress notes, physician's orders, previous consultations and any other pertinent information remaining in the patient's chart.

CHIEF COMPLAINT: Diabetic foot care

PHYSICAL EXAMINATION: The patient is a 57-year-old white male admitted with a history of hypertension and diabetes mellitus, insulin dependent for approximately 7 years. The patient has shortness of breath and is a smoker. The patient states that he has had a problem with one of the valves in his heart for approximately 3 years. The patient had resection of an aneurysm in the right leg in 1989. The patient has no known drug allergies. Multiple nails, right and left feet are hypertrophic and mycotic with in-growing tendencies. The patient has had trauma to both the great toenails at the age of 12 years due to a vehicular accident. Gait analysis will be deferred at this time. Pulses are present in both feet and ankles. The toes are warm. There are no digital lesions at this time. The muscle tone and power are fair. The patient denied having intermittent claudication during gait or phlebitis affecting either lower extremity. The patient does have some numbness of the right great toe, status post-surgery for the popliteal aneurysm.

IMPRESSION:

1. Type 1 diabetes mellitus
2. Congestive heart failure
3. Valvular heart disease
4. Smoker
5. Status post resection of aneurysm of the right leg
6. Hypertension

PLAN: Podiatric consultation; initial; comprehensive. Debridement of hypertrophic mycotic nail plates bilateral feet—symptomatic

PROCEDURE: Debridement of hypertrophic mycotic nail plates, bilateral feet, symptomatic

RECOMMENDATIONS: Diabetic foot care q. 1 to 3 months. The patient will be followed p.r.n.

PROGRESS NOTES—PATIENT 11

DATE	NOTE
1/27	Physical examination reveals rales and evidence of valvular heart disease. Will diurese with Lasix and obtain an echocardiogram.
1/28	Patient better today—no shortness of breath, no edema. The importance of smoking cessation was discussed with the patient.
1/29	Will discharge the patient today.

PHYSICIAN'S ORDERS—PATIENT 11

DATE	ORDER
1/27	Chest x-ray
	Monitor input and output
	Lasix 40 mg IV now and 40 mg PO in a.m.
	Schedule patient for an echocardiogram
	CBC
	Consult podiatry for diabetic foot care
	Lotensin 20 mg PO daily in a.m.
1/23	Discharge patient to home.

LABORATORY REPORTS—PATIENT 11

HEMATOLOGY

DATE: 1/27

Specimen	Results	Normal Values
WBC	10	4.3–11.0
RBC	5.0	4.5–5.9
HGB	16.2	13.5–17.5
HCT	48	41–52
MCV	93	80–100
MCHC	35	31–57
PLT	339	150–450

RADIOLOGY REPORT—PATIENT 11

DATE: 1/28

Chest x-ray

DIAGNOSIS: The examination is compared to a prior examination on March 2 of last year. The cardiac silhouette remains at the upper limits of normal in size. The pulmonary vascularity appears slightly congested and there is a right-sided pleural effusion that was not present on the prior examination. There is minimal blunting of the left costophrenic angle. The appearance suggests congestive heart failure.

IMPRESSION: Findings of congestive heart failure

Enter seven diagnosis codes and two procedure codes.

PDX

DX2

DX3

DX4

DX5

DX6

DX7

PP1

PR2

INPATIENT RECORD—PATIENT 12

DISCHARGE SUMMARY

DATE OF ADMISSION: 10/21   **DATE OF DISCHARGE:** 10/22

DISCHARGE DIAGNOSIS: Retained products of conception with vaginal bleeding following dilation and curettage (D & C) for miscarriage and tobacco and alcohol abuse.

COURSE IN HOSPITAL: The patient was admitted to the emergency department due to fainting and vaginal bleeding. The patient was taken to the OR for D & C. Pathology revealed decidua and chronic villa. She previously underwent a D & C for a miscarriage last week at another institution. The patient was encouraged to decrease her alcohol intake and to stop smoking. The patient appeared depressed over her recent miscarriage. A psych consult was ordered.

INSTRUCTIONS ON DISCHARGE: If heavy bleeding occurs, contact my office immediately. A follow-up visit is scheduled with the psychiatrist in 2 weeks. The patient was also given information about Alcoholics Anonymous as well as a prescription for Wellbutrin to be taken as directed for depression and smoking cessation.

HISTORY AND PHYSICAL EXAMINATION—PATIENT 12

ADMITTED: 10/21

REASON FOR ADMISSION: Heavy bleeding from vagina

HISTORY OF PRESENT ILLNESS: She has had irregular spotting and light flow on and off since a spontaneous abortion that occurred last week. She was admitted to another hospital at that time and underwent a D & C. The patient noted heavy bleeding today. She fainted in the bathroom and was brought to the emergency department by her family.

PAST MEDICAL HISTORY: The patient developed bronchitis as a child, but was not treated other than with decongestant. Her last menstrual period was 6 weeks ago.

ALLERGIES: None known

CHRONIC MEDICATIONS: None

FAMILY HISTORY: Mother has hypertension. Two sisters have had heart surgery for congenital heart problems.

SOCIAL HISTORY: The patient smokes one pack of cigarettes per day and reports intake of one 6-pack every few days during the week. The patient tried to abstain from alcohol during her pregnancy but was not successful.

REVIEW OF SYSTEMS: The patient is normally healthy. She has had a runny nose for about two days. Her bowel movements are normal, once every 2 to 3 days and her urinary function is normal. She eats three meals per day. She gets heartburn when she eats spicy foods. She drinks with her meals and into the evening on a continual basis.

HISTORY AND PHYSICAL EXAMINATION — PATIENT 12 (continued)

PHYSICAL EXAMINATION:

HEENT: PERRLA, EOM normal, thyroid not enlarged

CHEST: Clear to P & A without CVA tenderness

HEART: NSR without murmur

ABDOMEN: Soft and nontender with active bowel sounds

EXTREMITIES: Without edema, cyanosis, or clubbing

NEURO: CN's II–XII grossly intact. Reflexes are normal. No sensory or motor defects noted.

PELVIC: Uterus is of normal size with AV and femoral adnexa negative. Vaginal vault filled with serum fluid and clots. Cervix reveals pink with blood oozing from OS—no foreign body or laceration noted.

ASSESSMENT: Dysfunctional uterine bleeding

PLAN: D & C

CONSULTATION — PATIENT 12

PSYCH CONSULT

Thank you for requesting a consult with this patient. I met with her and found her to be depressed secondary to recent miscarriage. There was no evidence of suicidal thoughts. She denies any thoughts of harming herself or others. The patient has a history of alcohol abuse, three 6-packs of beer per week, and tobacco 1 ppd.

IMPRESSION:

1. Depression—secondary to recent miscarriage

2. Alcohol abuse

3. Tobacco abuse

Will treat with Wellbutrin 150 mg PO daily × 3 days then BID thereafter. Follow up in 2 weeks.

PROGRESS NOTES—PATIENT 12

DATE	NOTE
10/21	The patient has been bleeding for approximately 1 week utilizing at least 3 pads per day for flow of blood. We will repeat the D & C to determine if the patient has retained products of conception.

PREOPERATIVE DIAGNOSIS: Severe menorrhagia

POSTOPERATIVE DIAGNOSIS: Same

OPERATION: Dilatation and curettage

ANESTHESIA: Paracervical block using 1% Xylocaine and sedation using IV Valium

The patient tolerated the procedure well. Await pathology report.

The patient appears depressed, will order a psych consult.

DATE	NOTE
10/22	The patient has decreased bleeding with decreased cramping. Will discharge today. Psych consult appreciated. The importance of decreasing alcohol and tobacco use was stressed as was the effect of these substances on fetal development. The patient will follow up with the psychiatrist after discharge.

PHYSICIAN'S ORDERS—PATIENT 12

DATE	ORDER
10/21	Admit the patient to the labor and delivery floor
	Vaginal prep
	1,000 cc LR
	NPO
	Type and screen
	CBC
	Psych consult
10/22	Discharge patient to home

OPERATIVE REPORT—PATIENT 12

DATE: 10/21

PREOPERATIVE DIAGNOSIS: Severe menorrhagia

POSTOPERATIVE DIAGNOSIS: Same

OPERATION: Dilatation and curettage

ANESTHESIA: Paracervical block using 1% Xylocaine and sedation using IV Valium

OPERATIVE PROCEDURE: The patient was brought to the operating room and placed in the supine position. After IV Valium sedation, the patient was placed in the lithotomy position. The vaginal and perineal areas were then prepped and draped in the usual manner for vaginal surgery. Weighted speculum was inserted and the anterior retractor was used to expose the cervix. The cervix was then grasped using the Jacob's tenaculum. The paracervical block was then performed and then using Pratt dilators, the cervix was dilated up to #23. The uterus was then sounded and found to be approximately 7.5 cm. Using a medium-sized sharp curette, the uterine cavity was then curetted in systematic fashion from 12 o'clock clockwise to 6 o'clock and then from 12 o'clock counterclockwise to 6 o'clock. Endometrial tissue obtained was sent to pathology. The Jacob's tenaculum was removed and with assurance of hemostasis, the weighted speculum was removed. The patient tolerated the procedure and anesthesia well and arrived in the recovery room in satisfactory condition.

PATHOLOGY REPORT—PATIENT 12

DATE: 10/22

GROSS DESCRIPTION: Labeled "endometrium" are multiple irregular fragments of tan-white tissue and blood clots, forming a spheroid 1.0 cm in diameter. All blocked.

MICROSCOPIC DESCRIPTION:

DIAGNOSIS: Secretory endometrium, with necrotic fragments of decidua and chorionic villi, consistent with retained products of conception.

LABORATORY REPORTS—PATIENT 12

HEMATOLOGY

DATE: 10/21

Specimen	Results	Normal Values
WBC	10	4.3–11.0
RBC	5.0	4.5–5.9
HGB	13.5	13.5–17.5
HCT	41	41–52
MCV	93	80–100
MCHC	35	31–57
PLT	339	150–450

Enter five diagnosis codes and one procedure code.

PDX

DX2

DX3

DX4

DX5

PP1

Answer Key

CCS

Introduction

Case-Mix Exercise

1. The pyelonephritis (590.80) has a weight of 0.7870 whereas dehydration (276.51) has a weight of 0.6988. In this case, the pyelonephritis used as principal results in a higher-paying MS-DRG. This is appropriate based on the coding guideline II.C: *Two or more diagnoses that equally meet the definition for principal diagnosis* (Brown 2012, 29).

2. Using the pneumonia code first in sequence (486) has a weight of 0.7037 whereas congestive heart failure (428.0) has a weight of 1.5010. The MS-DRG 0291, HEART FAILURE & SHOCK W MCC has a higher weight (Medicare Grouper Version 29-10/11).

3. *Escherichia coli* pneumonia (482.82) has a weight of 1.4653 whereas COPD with acute exacerbation (491.21) has a weight of 01.1684. The bacterial pneumonia MS-DRG has a higher weight (Medicare Grouper Version 28-10/11).

4. CM = 0.7870 + 1.5010 + 1.4653 = 3.7533, CMI = 3.7533 / 3 = 1.2511. The case mix can be determined by multiplying the relative weight of each MS-DRG by the number of discharges within that MS-DRG. The sum of all the weights is the case mix. Dividing the case mix by the total number of MS-DRGs is the case-mix index (LaTour and Eichenwald Maki 2010, 436).

E/M Mapping Exercise

1. Diagnosis: 786.59, 305.1 (HHS 2011, Section IV, H).

2. CPT code using map 1—no meds given (5 points), history is PF (10 points), examination is EPF (15), tests are 5 (15 points), and supplies are none (points equal 0). Total points = 45. There were both radiology and lab tests done. CPT is 99283–25. The mapping method would be used and every hospital can develop a unique method (Clark 2009, 72–73).

Coding Exercises

Inpatient

1. 550.90, 042, 53.02 (Schraffenberger 2012, 82–84, 235–236).

2. 276.51, 438.82, 787.20 (Schraffenberger 2012, 125–127, 198–199).

3. 303.00, 571.2, 305.40, 94.68 (Schraffenberger 2012, 146–148).

4. 345.90, 350.1 (Schraffenberger 2012, 161–162).

5. 486,427.31—In accordance with the UHDDS, both conditions are not equally treated. The pneumonia was treated with IV antibiotics. This diagnosis had greater utilization of resources of medications and staff time compared with the atrial fibrillation, which was treated with oral medication. Because of this, the pneumonia is sequenced first (HHS 2011, Section II, C).

6. 574.10, 575.8, V64.41, 51.22 (Schraffenberger 2012, 454; HHS 2011, Section I, 18. d, 14).

7. 592.0, 591, 56.0 (Brown 2012, 224).

8. 707.07, 715.36, 707.20, 86.22 (Schraffenberger 2012, 293–294, 297).

9. 722.10, 80.51 (Schraffenberger 2012, 305).

10a. 656.61, 666.02, V27.0, 72.1—The patient had a hemorrhage that occurred after delivery but before the expulsion of the placenta. This hemorrhage, by definition, occurred in the third stage of labor. The patient has delivered and therefore assign a fifth digit of 2, which is why 666.02 was assigned. (Schraffenberger 2012, 270, 278–283).

10b. V30.00 (Schraffenberger 2012, 443–444).

11. V32.01, 765.14, 773.1, 765.26 (Schraffenberger 2012, 243–244, 325–326).

12. 414.01, 411.1, 37.22, 88.57—The clinical scenario is one typical of unstable angina (*Coding Clinic* 5th issue, 1993, 17–24). Coronary artery disease is coded as principal (*Coding Clinic* 2nd Quarter 2004, 3; Schraffenberger 2012, 189–190).

13. 162.5, 198.3, 32.49 (Schraffenberger 2012, 102).

14. 198.5, 199.1 (Schraffenberger 2012, 108–109).

15. 197.7, V10.3, V45.71 (Schraffenberger 2012, 437, 445–446).

16. 823.31, 822.0, 79.26 (Schraffenberger 2012, 354–355).

17. 969.4, 963.0, 780.2, E853.2, E858.1—The patient took over-the-counter medications with a prescription medication without consulting the prescribing physician. This is a poisoning. Per the *Official ICD-9-CM Guidelines for Coding and Reporting*, I, C, 17, e, 2, c: Nonprescribed drug taken with correctly prescribed and properly administered drug: If a nonprescribed drug or medicinal agent was taken in combination with a correctly prescribed and properly administered drug, any drug toxicity or other reaction resulting from the interaction of the two drugs would be classified as a poisoning (*Coding Clinic* 2nd Quarter 2002; HHS 2011, Section I, 17, e; Schraffenberger 2012, 382–384).

18. 996.64, 038.11, 995.91 (Brown 2012, 80–81, 386).

19. ICD: 769; 31.1 (Schraffenberger 2012 386, 80–81; *Coding Clinic* 1986 Nov.–Dec., 6; 1st Quarter 1989, 10).

Ambulatory/Outpatient

20. ICD: 786.59; CPT: 91034 (Schraffenberger 2012, 338–340; *CPT Assistant* May 2005, 3).

21. ICD: V76.12; CPT: 77057 (*Coding Clinic* 2nd Quarter 2003, 3–5; 2nd Quarter 2005, 2010; *CPT Assistant* March 2007, 7).

22. ICD: 173.11; CPT: 11642 (Schraffenberger 2012, 94–102; *CPT Assistant* Fall 1995, 3; May 1996,11; Feb. 2008, 8; Feb. 2010, 3; *CPT Changes: An Insider's View 2003*).

23. ICD: 735.0; CPT: 28293–TA (Schraffenberger 2012, 305; *CPT Assistant* Dec. 1996, 6; *CPT Assistant* Jan. 2007, 31).

24. ICD: 197.2 183.0; CPT: 32650 (Schraffenberger 2012, chapter 5; *CPT Assistant* Fall 1994, 1, 6; *CPT Changes: An Insider's View 2002*).

25. ICD: 427.81, 427.89; CPT: 33228 (Schraffenberger 2012, 194–195; *CPT Changes: An Insider's View 2003; CPT Assistant* Summer 1994, 10, 19; *CPT Assistant* Nov. 1999, 16; *CPT Changes: An Insider's View* 2000, 2012).

26. ICD: 456.1; CPT: 43243 (Schraffenberger 2012, 203; Smith 2013, 118; *CPT Assistant* Spring 1994, 4).

27. ICD: 600.00; CPT: 52601 (Schraffenberger 2012, 252; Smith 2013, 139; *CPT Assistant* Nov. 1997, 20; CPT Assistant April 2001, 4; *CPT Assistant* June 2003, 6).

28. ICD: 222.1; CPT: 54056 (Schraffenberger 2012, 103; Smith 2013, 139).

29. ICD: 626.8; CPT: 58563 (Schraffenberger 2012, chapter 13; *CPT Assistant* Nov. 1999, 28; March 2000, 10; March 2002, 11; *CPT Changes: An Insider's View* 2000, 2002).

30. ICD: 654.53; CPT: 59871 (Brown 2012, 278; *CPT Assistant* Nov. 1997, 22; *CPT Assistant* Nov. 2006, 21; *CPT Assistant* Feb. 2007, 10).

Practice

1. **c** The patient is discharged with hemiplegia and aphasia. These conditions in addition to the acute cerebral infarction should be coded (Brown 2012, chapter 24, *Coding Clinic* 4th Quarter 1998, Vol. 15(4): 87).

2. **b** When a patient has pulmonary edema that is due to congestive heart failure, only the congestive heart failure should be coded (Brown 2012, chapter 24, *Coding Clinic* 4th Quarter 2009, Vol. 26).

3. **b** The CPK elevation with MB enzymes elevated and the EKG ST changes denote a possible MI (Brown 2012, chapter 24).

4. **d** Symptoms are not coded when a definitive diagnosis is present on discharge. The patient has a discharge diagnosis of urinary tract infection. The organism (*E. coli*) is coded with a secondary diagnosis code (041.49) which is to be added as an additional code to identify the bacterial agent (*Coding Clinic* 1st Quarter 1998, 5; *Coding Clinic* July–August 1984, 19).

5. **a** When the documentation is not clear regarding a potential complication, it is appropriate to query the physician (Brown 2012, chapter 4).

6. **b** The symptoms provided are indicative of a depressive disorder (Brown 2012, 137).

7. **c** The patient has abdominal adhesions with obstruction, and lysis of adhesions was performed. The abdominal pain is not coded as it is a symptom (*Coding Clinic* Nov.–Dec. 1987; *Coding Clinic* Jan.–Feb. 1987; *Coding Clinic* 4th Quarter 1990, 18–19; *Coding Clinic* 3rd Quarter 1995, 6; *Coding Clinic* 4th Quarter 1995, 55; Brown 2012, 208). Code 997.49, postoperative digestive system complications, excludes peritoneal (abdominal) adhesions codes 568.0 and code 568.81. In the Alphabetic Index, under Adhesions, postoperative, you will also find that 568.0 is used. Because of this, assign 568.81 for abdominal adhesions with obstruction.

8. **c** Patient is found to have dysphagia with aspiration is the correct answer because it changes the coding to aspiration pneumonia and would result in MS-DRG 179 RESPIRATORY INFECTIONS & INFLAMMATIONS W/O CC/MCC MDC, which has a weight of 01.0025 (Medicare Grouper Version Used: 29-10/11). This is in comparison to MS-DRG 0195, SIMPLE PNEUMONIA & PLEURISY W/O CC/MCC MDC: 04 which has a DRG weight of 00.7037 (Medicare Grouper Version Used: 29-10/11).

9. **d**   There may be endometrial implants throughout the pelvic cavity which may attach to various anatomic structures such as the fallopian tube, ovary, and omentum. These locations should be identified so that the appropriate diagnostic codes can be assigned and the appropriate procedure codes can be assigned based on the destruction of the endometrial implants. Therefore, the correct answer is to review the operative report to determine what procedure codes to use and determine the site or sites of endometriosis so that codes with the highest specificity may be assigned. Also, use the diagnosis of infertility as a secondary condition (*Coding Clinic* 1st Quarter 1995; *CPT Assistant* 1999; *Coding Clinic* March 2000; Schraffenberger 2012, chapter 13; Brown 2012, 227).

10. **d**   The care rendered to the patient and the patient's response must be documented in the medical record (LaTour and Eichenwald Maki 2010, 213).

11. **b**   In order to prove authorship of documents they are required to be authenticated by a signature (LaTour and Eichenwald Maki 2010, 213).

12. **c**   The medical staff bylaws are required by accreditation and regulatory organizations to refer to the timeline required for completion (LaTour and Eichenwald Maki 2010, 214).

13. **a**   Poisoning codes for aspirin and heparin and subcutaneous hemorrhage of the thigh of the right lower extremity as secondary conditions. This is considered a poisoning because the patient took an over-the-counter (OTC) medication (aspirin) without consulting the clinical providers of a prescribed medication. Taking an OTC with a prescription medication is a criterion of poisoning. The poisoning codes are sequenced first before the manifestation codes (Brown 2012, 443–444; HHS 2011, Section I, 17, e, 2; *Coding Clinic* 4th Quarter 1995). Review Coding Guideline I, C, 17, e, 2, c for additional information.

14. **c**   Code 996.01 pertains to mechanical complications and would not be used. In this case, there is pain due to the electrode. Category 996.7 is the location for pain due to devices. Under the heading of 996.7 in the Tabular Index you will find the list of what is covered in this category. The breast cyst (610.0) would not be coded because it does not meet the criteria of the UHDDS as a secondary condition; it is an incidental finding (Brown 2012, 30–33). Code V45.79 is not added as an additional diagnosis. Review the Alphabetic Index under Absence, thyroid, with hypothyroidism, which directs the coder to code 244.0.

15. **b**   The abdominal pain and diarrhea are not coded as they are symptoms integral to the diagnosis of infectious gastroenteritis (Brown 2012, chapter 9).

16. **c**   The circumstances of the encounter are for a screening colonoscopy. Because of this the screening, colonoscopy is listed first, followed by a code for the polyps (*Coding Clinic* 2nd Quarter 2005, 16–17).

17. **a**   The Includes notes direct what types of neoplasms should be assigned to category 216 (Brown 2012, 17). Includes notes in category 216 specify the use of these codes (HHS 2011).

18. **b**   The Excludes notes direct what types of neoplasms should not be assigned to category 216 (Brown 2012, 17–18). Excludes notes in category 216 specify the use of these codes (HHS 2011).

19. **b**   The patient has mature senile cataracts, diabetes mellitus (with no designated causal relationship to the cataracts), hypertension, acute renal failure. The hypertension is not related to the renal failure as it is acute and not chronic. Because of this, a combination code for hypertension and chronic renal failure is not coded (*Coding Clinic* 3rd Quarter 1991; *Coding Clinic* 2nd Quarter 1992; Brown 2012, 123–126, 172, 221).

20. **d** Acute exacerbation is coded as 491.21. The hypertension is present with the chronic renal disease. Because of this, a combination code for hypertension and chronic renal disease is coded. In addition, the type of kidney disease and stage are coded (Brown 2012, 186–188, 220–222; *Coding Clinic* 4th Quarter 2006).

21. **a** The patient was admitted and treated for the respiratory failure. The other conditions present are also coded (Brown 2012, 189–191; *Coding Clinic* 1st Quarter 2005).

22. **d** The patient has cirrhosis of the liver with resulting bleeding esophageal varices. Under subcategory 456.2, see the note *Code first underlying cause, as:* Cirrhosis of liver (571.0–571.9). Because of this note, the cirrhosis is sequenced first followed by the code for the bleeding esophageal varices, followed by the code for the bleeding esophageal varices (Brown 2012, 203; *Coding Clinic* May–June 1984).

23. **b** The physician may word the delivery as "normal" but the coder cannot use 650 unless the patient meets the criteria for using it. The patient has a nuchal cord around the baby's neck which precludes the use of 650 (HHS 2011, Section I, C, 11; Brown 2012, chapter 20).

24. **c** Codes must reflect the twin gestation as well as early delivery (Brown 2012, chapter 20).

25. **a** The ulcerative colitis and osteoporosis should be coded as well as the adverse effect and long term use of the steroid (Schraffenberger 2012, 236, 377, 450).

26. **d** In order to determine the correct procedure code the lengths of the wounds repaired with the same closure are added together (AMA 2013, Surgery/Integumentary Section directions).

27. **d** The patient has a fracture of the right proximal ulna and closed reduction is necessary. In the *ICD-9-CM* codebook, under Fracture, ulna, proximal, the coder is referred to Fracture, ulna, upper end. The term "manipulation" is used to indicate reduction in CPT (AMA 2013, 123).

28. **b** A code for the anterior ethmoidectomy is assigned and to denote the bilateral procedure, a modifier of –50 is added (*CPT Assistant* Winter 1993, 23; Jan. 1997, 4; Sept. 1997, 10; Oct. 1997, 5; Dec. 2001, 6; May 2003, 5). The sinusotomy is not coded separately, as it is a diagnostic procedure.

29. **c** In contrast to question 28, the code description for the transbronchial biopsy includes the specification that the biopsy is in a single lobe. An additional CPT code is needed (as opposed to a modifier) to denote the bilateral aspect of the biopsy. CPT code 31632 is an "add-on" code, which means it is coded in addition to the primary procedure code (AMA 2013, 161-163; *CPT Assistant* 2005; May 2008, 15; Feb. 2010, 6; April 2010, 5).

30. **b** There is a combination code for a left and right cardiac catheterization (37.23). Both the diagnostic cardiac catheterization and the cardiac angiography procedures are assigned (Brown 2012, 356; *Coding Clinic* 2nd Quarter 2005, 10–11).

31. **a** The procedure code assigned is associated with the diagnosis of missed abortion (Brown 2012, 300; *Coding Clinic* 3rd Quarter 1993, 6).

32. **b** Modifier –50 would not be used as this modifier pertains to paired organs only (*CPT Assistant* Feb. 2000, 4; Nov. 2008, 11; Oct. 2009, 12).

33. **c** Both the extraction of the cataract and the insertion of the lens are included in the single CPT code. The –RT modifier should be used to indicate the right eye was involved (*CPT Assistant* Nov. 2003, 10; March 2005, 11; Sept. 2009, 5).

34. **a** Three codes are needed to capture the initial hour and the two additional hours. Modifier –51 would not be used in this case because modifiers are not used with add-on codes (96415) (*CPT Assistant* Nov. 2005, 1; Jan. 2007, 3; May 2007, 3; Sept. 2007, 3; Dec. 2007, 15; Feb. 2009, 17).

35. **b** The code for a complete chest x-ray includes a minimum of four views and does not include computer-aided detection or fluoroscopy (*CPT Assistant* July 2007, 6; Dec. 2009, 14).

36. **c** The localization and aspiration require two codes to identify both radiological guidance and the procedure itself (*CPT Assistant* March 2007, 7).

37. **b** The code that best fits the ligation is the fulguration because there are no clips or excision or lesion completed during the procedure (*CPT Assistant* Nov. 1999, 29; March 2000, 10).

38. **c** The type of cholecystectomy should be coded. In this case, it is a laparoscopic cholecystectomy (Brown 2012, 206).

39. **c** The fifth digit 1 is used to indicate the initial episode of care for the myocardial infarction. It is used for both Hospital A as well as Hospital B as the care for the acute infarction continued with the transfer to Hospital B for a definitive procedure (Brown 2012, chapter 24; *Coding Clinic* 4th Quarter 2007, 162–167; *Coding Clinic* 3rd Quarter 2007, 10).

40. **c** In the inpatient setting, "Rule Out" diagnoses are coded as if they exist. In this case the patient has chest pain and the reason for the chest pain is rule our gastroesophageal reflux disease (GERD). This requires that the GERD be coded as the first listed diagnosis (Brown 2012, 57).

41. **d** The ventilator management is the procedure that will impact the MS-DRG to provide appropriate reimbursement. The MS-DRG with the highest weight is 870 (Medicare Grouper Version 29-10/11).

    Ventilator management for 106 consecutive hours (96.72). Medicare DRG assigned: 0870, SEPTICEMIA OR SEVERE SEPSIS W MV 96+ HOURS DRG weight = 05.8339.

    Incorrect answer option explanations provided for clarity:

    a. Bronchoscopy with biopsy (33.24) reference: Medicare DRG assigned: 872 SEPTICEMIA OR SEVERE SEPSIS W/O MV 96+ HOURS W/O MCC MDC: 18 DRG weight = 01.1339 (*incorrect*)

    b. Debridement of nails (86.27) reference: Medicare DRG assigned: 872 SEPTICEMIA OR SEVERE SEPSIS W/O MV 96+ HOURS W/O MCC MDC: 18 DRG weight = 01.1339 (*incorrect*)

    c. Nonexcisional debridement of skin ulcer with abrasion (86.28) reference: Medicare DRG assigned: 872 SEPTICEMIA OR SEVERE SEPSIS W/O MV 96+ HOURS W/O MCC MDC: 18 DRG weight = 01.1339 (*incorrect*)

42. **c** Metastatic carcinoma of the brain; history of carcinoma of the prostate. The patient does not have a current cancer of the prostate however is being admitted and treated for metastatic cancer (to the brain, from the prostate) (HHS 2011, Section I, C, 2, b).

43. **a** The conditions residual effects that the patient has been discharged with are coded in addition to the cerebral infarction. For code 342.91, the fifth digit 1 is used to identify the infarction and hemiplegia is on the left side of the brain which affects the right side of the body in this right-handed patient (Brown 2012, chapter 24).

44. **c** The diagnosis after study (lung cancer) was present on admission as well as the symptom (hemoptysis). Code 770.3 would not be assigned because it is not diagnosed and only applies to the perinatal period (Brown 2012, Appendix A; HHS 2011, Appendix 1).

45. **b** Policies and procedures of the medical staff are not relevant. But the other areas of diagnoses, additional conditions, and procedures are all important to determine the MS-DRG (Brown 2012, 35).

46. **b** While Medicare may specify that a given condition is not acceptable, if that condition is what is documented the coder has no other option but to code what is documented even though the insurer may not pay the claim (Brown 2012, 35).

47. **c** It is important to understand the time frame for assigning a status code specifying that a condition is present on admission (Brown 2012, 451).

48. **a** The physician must establish the diagnosis—obesity or morbid obesity—and the additional information can be pulled from ancillary documentation to establish the correct code assignment, for body mass index (BMI) (Brown 2012, 541).

49. **c** The surgery is done on two distinct body systems with two distinct approaches. This warrants the use of –59 (*CPT Assistant* Sept. 2001).

50. **d** Because the lungs are paired organs, it may seem as though modifier -50 would be appropriate. However, a modifier would not be assigned because the bronchus is not a paired organ, and the bronchus is the location of the procedure, not the lungs. In order to assign the correct modifier, it is important to note that paired organs include ears, eyes, nostrils, kidneys, lungs, ovaries, and such. (*CPT Assistant* May 2003).

51. **c** The melanoma is coded to the site of the lesion and the procedure code is determined based on the size of the lesion as well as the margins excised (Brown 2012, chapter 25; *CPT Assistant* Fall 1995, 3; May 1996, 11; Nov. 2002, 5; Feb. 2010, 3).

52. **b** The bleeding is included in the code for diverticulosis and therefore a second code is not warranted (*CPT Assistant* 4th Quarter 1990, 20–24).

53. **c** The patient has a recurrent hernia without obstruction and this is captured in diagnosis code 550.91 (Brown 2012, chapter 16; *CPT Assistant* Nov. 1999, 24; March 2000, 9).

54. **d** The fracture code also includes the time of unconsciousness. The E code is provided here as part of the review; however, no E codes are used on the exam except those for poisonings and adverse effects of drugs (Brown 2012, chapters 8 and 26). (Based on inpatient exam instructions, do not code procedures that fall within the code range 87.01–99.99 unless the code is listed in the instructions. 87.07 is not listed. Also see the Procedures for Coding Medical Record Cases for the CCS Examination in the Introduction of this book.)

55. **c** The principal diagnosis requires that the condition after study, which occasioned the patient's admission to the hospital, be assigned as the principal diagnosis. In the outpatient setting, no after study element is involved as continued evaluation cannot occur (Brown 2012, 34).

56. **b** Surgical procedure names can be similar and it is important to have reference books in which to look up procedures in order to determine reportable and nonreportable procedures (Smith 2012, 36).

57. **b** This final rule established APCs by dividing outpatient services into fixed-payment groups (Smith 2013, 261).

58. **d** The code editor software reviews many data elements and compares them to what data specifications are required in order to weed out incomplete or incorrect claims (Smith 2013, 266).

59. **c** There isn't a combination code for acute renal failure and hypertension. Acute kidney failure is not the same as chronic kidney disease (Brown 2012, 220–221).

60. **d** Per *CPT Assistant*, "Codes 52234–52240 should only be reported once, regardless of the number of tumors removed. Only one of the three codes may be reported per session. Select the code based on the largest tumor. Note that 52234 is used when one or more of the tumors is from 0.5 cm to 2.0 cm. Code 52240 is used when one or more of the tumors are larger than 5.0 cm" (AMA August 2009, 6).

61. **d** Both are types of prospective payment systems (CMS 2008).

62. **c** $10 \times 2.0 + 10 \times 1.5 + 10 \times 1.0 / 30 = 1.5$ The case mix can be determined by multiplying the relative weight of each MS-DRG by the number of discharges within that MS-DRG. The sum of all the weights is the case mix. Dividing the case mix by the total number of MS-DRGs is the case-mix index (LaTour and Eichenwald Maki 2010, 436).

63. **a** The MS-DRG weight is higher than the other MS-DRG weights and therefore the associated MS-DRG pays the most (Johns 2011, 323).

64. **b** Data quality may have slightly different meanings because there are several disciplines that work with data in healthcare. Generally, ensuring the accuracy and completeness of an organization's data is a definition that can be agreed upon by the organization (LaTour and Eichenwald Maki 2010, 963).

65. **d** A good process to ensure the data is accurate is to make certain each record or entry within the database is correct (LaTour and Eichenwald Maki 2010, 120).

66. **a** There are many characteristics of data but in terms of timeliness, a patient's medications being available for patient care is an important example (LaTour and Eichenwald Maki 2010, 125).

67. **d** Data can only be identified as high-quality when they conform to a recognized standard (LaTour and Eichenwald Maki 2010, 117).

68. **a** The cancer registry can be used to undertake studies in addition to reporting cases to a central registry (LaTour and Eichenwald Maki 2010, 333).

69. **c** The diagnostic index can be used with the cancer registry data to undertake data quality analysis (LaTour and Eichenwald Maki 2010, 331–333).

70. **a** Several data sources can assist the process of improving data quality in this scenario (LaTour and Eichenwald Maki 2010, chapter 12).

71. **d**   There are many types of diagrams but one that depicts a relational database structure is an entity diagram (LaTour and Eichenwald Maki 2010, 128).

72. **a**   There are several definitions of mapping and crosswalks but an important one in healthcare is that they are used to describe paths between classifications and vocabularies (LaTour and Eichenwald Maki 2010, 131).

73. **c**   Object-oriented databases are becoming increasingly common. The unique quality of these databases is that data and their relationships are specified within a single structure (LaTour and Eichenwald Maki 2010, 128).

74. **d**   Structured query language (SQL) is used commonly for data language and data definitions (LaTour and Eichenwald Maki 2010, 127).

75. **a**   Only records that are required for care or authorized by the patient can be released by the urgent-care facility to the acute-care facility (LaTour and Eichenwald Maki 2010, chapter 10).

76. **d**   Only conditions or procedures that are supported by documentation can be coded (LaTour and Eichenwald Maki 2010, chapter 11).

77. **d**   Disclosing information without the patient's written consent violates the patient's right to privacy (LaTour and Eichenwald Maki 2010, chapter 10).

78. **d**   Health information should not be left in public view (LaTour and Eichenwald Maki 2010, chapter 10).

79. **d**   Only those conditions that are documented by the physician should be coded (LaTour and Eichenwald Maki 2010, chapter 11).

80. **d**   If a procedure is performed, the operative report provides a detailed discussion of what was done (LaTour and Eichenwald Maki 2010, chapter 10).

81. **b**   In order to code the procedure accurately, specific information must be documented and used to assign the code (Brown 2012, chapter 24).

82. **b, c, f**   The Tabular Index directs the coder to code both the hypertensive heart disease and stage V kidney disease as well as a code for the congestive heart failure and the chronic kidney disease, stage V (Brown 2012, 348–349).

83. **c, d, e**   Code the CHF as well as hypertension with end stage kidney disease. In this exercise, both hypertension and chronic kidney disease are documented and for this reason code a combination code. The combination code for hypertensive heart disease is not used in this case as a causal relationship between the hypertension and the CHF was not documented (Brown 2012, 339, 348).

84. **a, d, f**   Code the hypertension with stage III chronic kidney disease. In this case both hypertension and chronic kidney disease are documented and a combination code is used. Also the code for the stage III chronic kidney disease must be assigned due to the "code also" note. The acute renal failure is identified with a separate code (Brown 2012, 220–221, 348).

85. **b, c**   There is a cause and effect relationship established between the hypertension and the congestive heart failure. A separate code for the congestive heart failure is assigned based on the "code also" note. (Brown 2012, 348).

86. **a, b, e**   The surgical package refers to a combination of individual services provided during one surgical operation (Smith 2013, 54).

87. **a**   When a procedure is designated as a separate procedure in the CPT codebook and it is performed in conjunction with another service, it is considered an integral part of the major service. The CPT code description includes "separate procedure." The intention is not to provide payment for a procedure that is already integral to a any given procedure (AMA 2013, 58; Smith 2013, 56).

88. **c, e, f**   When an question is asked about an outpatient acuity map, the coder must review the map and determine the relevant elements that make up the means by which a CPT code and level is assigned. In the case of this map these elements are specified as being important to determine the acuity points: number of tests ordered, supplies used, and medications are the key elements. Extent of history and extent of exam are important too but they are not listed in the multiple choice answer options.

89. **b, d, f**   The answers to these three questions must be known in order to code repairs correctly (AMA 2013,70-71; Smith 2013, 67).

PRACTICE—PATIENT 1

PDX	550.90	Inguinal hernia, without mention of obstruction or gangrene, unilateral or unspecified (not specified as recurrent)
DX2	214.4	Lipoma of spermatic cord (as per path. and operative reports)
PP1	49505–LT	Repair initial inguinal hernia, age 5 years or older; reducible
PR2	55520–59	Excision of lesion of spermatic cord (separate procedure)

Notes for Practice Outpatient Case—Patient 1

550.90   The type of hernia is coded (Brown 2012, 208–209).

214.4   The lipoma is also removed and so should be coded (Brown 2012, 377–378).

49505–LT   The hernia location is on the left and the laterality is reported (*CPT Assistant* Sept. 2000, 10).

55520–59   The lipoma requires excision and is therefore coded (*CPT Assistant* Sept. 2000, 10; Oct. 2001, 8).

PRACTICE — PATIENT 2

PDX	338.4	Chronic pain syndrome
DX2	724.4	Lumbar radiculopathy
PP1	62311	Injections(s), of diagnostic or therapeutic substance(s) (including anesthetic, antispasmodic, opioid, steroid, other solution), not including neurolytic substances, including needle or catheter placement, includes contrast for localization when performed, epidural or subarachnoid; lumbar or sacral (caudal)

Notes for Practice Outpatient Case—Patient 2

338.4   The patient has a diagnosis of chronic pain syndrome and a code from the 338 category should be assigned. Per the *Official ICD-9-CM Guidelines for Coding and Reporting* I, C, 6, 1, a: "Category 338 codes as principal or first-listed diagnosis." Category 338 codes are acceptable as principal diagnosis or the first-listed code when pain control or pain management is the reason for the admission/encounter. The underlying cause of the pain should be reported as an additional diagnosis, if known (Brown 2012, 163; *Coding Clinic* 2nd Quarter 2007, 14).

724.4   This code denotes the specific cause of the pain (Brown 2012, chapter 14).

62311   *CPT Assistant* states "62311 should only be coded once." This code is used for epidural injections (AMA Nov. 2008).

PRACTICE — PATIENT 3

PDX	338.3	Neoplasm related pain (acute) (chronic)
DX2	174.8	Malignant neoplasm of female breast, other specified sites
DX3	198.5	Secondary malignant neoplasm of bone and bone marrow
PP1	62362	Implantation or replacement of device for intrathecal or epidural drug infusion; programmable pump, including preparation of pump, with or without programming

Notes for Practice Outpatient Case—Patient 3

338.3   The patient is admitted for pain management due to metastatic cancer. If the admission is for pain control related to, associated with, or due to, a malignancy, code 338.3 (Brown 2012, 163; *Coding Clinic* 2nd Quarter 2007, 13–14).

174.8, 198.5   The primary site and metastatic (secondary) sites should be coded (Brown 2012, 378–382).

62362   The reservoir is surgically placed and attached to a previously placed catheter (*CPT Assistant* March 1997, 11).

PRACTICE—PATIENT 4

PDX	337.22	Reflex sympathetic dystrophy of the lower limb
PP1	64520–LT	Injection, anesthetic agent; lumbar or thoracic (paravertebral sympathetic)
PR2	77003	Fluoroscopic guidance and localization of needle or catheter tip for spine or paraspinous diagnostic or therapeutic injection procedures (epidural or subarachnoid)

Notes for Practice Outpatient Case—Patient 4

337.22   The diagnostic code is needed to establish the medical necessity for the procedure and a pain management code is not appropriate because the underlying condition is being treated (Brown 2012, 163).

64520–LT   When coding paravertebral spinal nerves and branches, it is appropriate to use the modifiers to note the laterality (*CPT Assistant* July 1998, 10; April 2005, 13).

77003   Fluoroscopic guidance is not included in the 64520 code so it is therefore appropriate to code a second code (*CPT Assistant* March 2007, 7; July 2008, 9; Feb. 2010, 12).

PRACTICE—PATIENT 5

PDX	182.0	Malignant neoplasm of body of uterus, corpus uteri, except isthmus
DX2	998.2	Accidental puncture or laceration during a procedure
DX3	998.09	Postoperative shock, other
DX4	285.1	Acute posthemorrhagic anemia
DX5	280.0	Iron deficiency anemia secondary to blood loss (chronic)
DX6	244.0	Postsurgical hypothyroidism
DX7	998.11	Hemorrhage complicating a procedure
DX8	568.81	Hemoperitoneum (nontraumatic)
DX9	V16.0	Family history of gastrointestinal tract
PP1	68.51	Laparoscopically assisted vaginal hysterectomy (LAVH)
PR2	39.31	Suture of artery

Notes for Practice Inpatient Case—Patient 5

182.0	Endometrial carcinoma is documented in the pathology report and the discharge summary (Brown 2012, 379–382).
998.2	Accidental laceration is documented in the second operative report (Brown 2012, 462). In the 998 category, a coder may double code—one code to denote the complication and the other to provide specificity. In other instances, only one code is needed. 998.2 is a general complication code. Adding an additional code notes what organ was lacerated.
998.09	Postoperative shock is denoted in the discharge summary (Brown 2012, 462). Include this because there is no other code to denote postoperative shock. Only one code is used. This is a new code for fiscal year 2012.
285.1	Acute blood loss anemia is documented in the progress notes and operative report because the patient had blood loss of 1,500 to 2,000 ml. The labs also reflect this diagnosis (*Coding Clinic* 2nd Quarter 1992).
280.0	The patient also had chronic blood loss anemia as documented on the H & P (*Coding Clinic* 4th Quarter 1993).
244.0	Postsurgical hypothyroidism is documented on the H & P report and patient received Synthroid while an inpatient (Brown 2012, 132).
998.11	Intraoperative hemorrhage documented in the operative report (Brown 2012, 462). 998.11 is a general complication code; the coder does not know where the hemorrhage is taking place. By adding an additional code, a coder can indicate where the hemorrhage is occurring.
568.81	Coded to add further specificity (Brown 2012, 453).
68.51	The patient underwent a laparoscopic-assisted vaginal hysterectomy. (Do not code the laparoscopy because it is the operative approach.) (Brown 2012, 68).
39.31	The patient underwent another laparoscopy for suture of the lacerated epigastric artery. (Do not code the laparoscopy because it is the operative approach.) (Brown 2012, 68).
Note:	Chronic cervicitis is not coded because it is an incidental finding (Brown 2012, 99).

Note: Based on the following instructions for the CCS exam (refer to the Procedures for Coding Medical Record Cases for the CCS Examination in the Introduction of this book), the blood transfusion is not coded: Do not code procedures that fall within the code range 87.01–99.99. But, code procedures in the following ranges:

87.51–87.54	Cholangiograms
87.74, 87.76	Retrogrades, urinary systems
88.40–88.58	Arteriography and angiography
92.21–92.29	Radiation therapy
94.24–94.27	Psychiatric therapy
94.61–94.69	Alcohol/drug detoxification and rehabilitation
96.04	Insertion of endotracheal tube
96.56	Other lavage of bronchus and trachea
96.70–96.72	Mechanical ventilation
98.51–98.59	ESWL
99.25	Chemotherapy

PRACTICE — PATIENT 6

PDX	V58.11	Encounter for antineoplastic chemotherapy
DX2	197.6	Secondary malignant neoplasm of retroperitoneum and peritoneum
DX3	789.51	Malignant ascites
DX4	V10.05	Personal history of malignant neoplasm of large intestine
DX5	V44.3	Status colostomy
DX6	V16.0	Family history of malignant neoplasm of gastrointestinal tract
DX7	V15.3	History of radiation therapy
DX8	V15.82	History of tobacco use
DX9	V45.72	Acquired absence of intestine (large) (small)
PP1	99.25	Chemotherapy

Notes on Practice Inpatient Case—Patient 6

V58.11 — The patient is admitted for chemotherapy, as documented in the discharge summary and reflected in the physician orders (Brown 2012, 391).

197.6 — Carcinomatosis with malignant ascites from retro-peritoneum and peritoneum is documented on the discharge summary and H & P (Brown 2012, 384–387).

789.51 — The *ICD-9-CM* Tabular Index requires the malignancy be coded first (Brown 2012, 384–387).

V10.05 — The organ of origin (colon) has been removed; therefore, code the history of malignant neoplasm of the colon. Whenever there is a secondary neoplasm code, primary site must be designated either with a code for the primary site or a V code. If the primary site for the neoplasm is not known, use code 199.1 (Brown 2012, 385–386).

V44.3 — Status colostomy is reflected on the H & P (Brown 2012, 89).

V16.0 — Relevant to the patient's treatment and documented in the medical record (Brown 2012, 83–84).

V15.3 — This code indicates that the patient has a history of radiation therapy (Brown 2012, 83–84).

V15.82 — This code indicates that the patient has a history of tobacco use and this is relevant because the patient has cancer (Brown 2012, 83–84).

V45.72 — The documentation indicates that a colectomy was done to treat the patient's primary colon cancer.

99.25 — Per the Procedures for Coding Medical Record Cases for the CCS Examination, this code for chemotherapy would be assigned. (For exam coding instructions, refer to the Introduction of this book.)

Note: — Breast cyst is not coded because it does not meet UHDDS criteria.

Points of Interest on Practice Patient 6

1. This case illustrates several basic principles of coding neoplasms. First, the patient had the organ in which the carcinoma arose removed (organ of origin). Second, because a secondary site is being coded, the coder must code the primary site in some manner. Therefore, use a history of malignancy code (V10.06) to represent the primary site.

2. This case also illustrates that when the ascites is determined to have malignant cells in the fluid, the code for malignant ascites should be used. Under code 789.51, there is a "code first malignancy, such as . . ." which determines the sequencing of the diagnosis codes.

PRACTICE—PATIENT 7

PDX	038.42	Septicemia due to Escherichia coli (E. coli)
DX2	590.10	Acute pyelonephritis, without lesion of renal medullary necrosis
DX3	054.9	Herpes simplex without mention of complication
DX4	V09.0	Infection with microorganisms resistant to penicillins
DX5	305.1	Tobacco use disorder

Notes on Inpatient Practice Case—Patient 7

038.42   *E. coli* septicemia is documented on the culture and sensitivity as well as in the H & P. SIRS is not used here because septicemia is documented, versus sepsis. (Brown 2012, 109–112).

590.10   Acute pyelonephritis is also coded because this is where the septicemia began. Do not code the organism (*Coding Clinic* 4th Quarter 1988). It is already reflected in the septicemia code (Brown 2012, 217).

054.9   Herpes simplex is documented on the 9/8 progress notes and is treated (Brown 2012, chapter 10).

305.1   Tobacco abuse is treated and documented in the progress notes, H & P and D/C summary. This code does not require a fifth digit (HHS 2011, Tabular Index; Brown 2012, chapter 12).

V09.0   The organism is specified to be resistant to in the discharge summary and therefore designate that in the coding (Brown 2012, 113).

Note: The pyelogram performed on 9/8 is not coded because it is an unspecified pyelogram (refer to the Procedures for Coding Medical Record Cases for the CCS Examination in the Introduction of this book). A pyelogram is coded only if it is code 87.74 or 87.76 (Retrogrades, urinary systems).

Points of Interest on Patient 7

1. This case illustrates how an infection can begin in one organ system and then become systemic. This is why the same organism is in the urinary tract and the blood. As stated earlier, code both disorders (septicemia and pyelonephritis).

2. The organism causing the infection is resistant to penicillin and ampicillin. Only code resistance to a drug if the resistance is documented by the practitioner in the record. Do not code from the laboratory reports alone.

Practice Exam 1

1. **c**   The American Thoracic Society has defined status asthmaticus as an acute asthmatic attack in which the degree of bronchial obstruction is not relieved by the usual treatment, such as by epinephrine or aminophylline (*Coding Clinic* 4th Quarter 1988, 9–10).

2. **c**   Unfortunately, urosepsis is sometimes stated as the diagnosis even though the condition has progressed to a septicemia in which a localized urinary tract infection has entered the blood stream and become a generalized sepsis. The physician should be asked if the diagnosis of urosepsis is intended to mean (1) generalized sepsis (septicemia) caused by leakage of urine or toxic urine by products into the general vascular circulation, or (2) urine contaminated by bacteria, bacterial by products, or other toxic material but without other findings (Brown 2012, 110).

3. **b**   It is rare for only one coronary artery to be bypassed, and it is also fairly common to perform both an internal mammary-coronary artery bypass and an aortocoronary bypass at the same operative episode (Schraffenberger 2012, 203–204).

4. **c**   A colonoscopy is an examination of the entire colon, from the rectum to the cecum that may include the terminal ileum. In general, a colonoscopy examines the colon to a level of 60 cm or higher (Smith 2013, 120).

5. **c**   Herceptin therapy is not antineoplastic chemotherapy, but is a biological adjuvant treatment for women with breast cancers that are HER2 positive. Herceptin is a type of targeted cancer therapy also referred to as a monoclonal antibody (*Coding Clinic* 3rd Quarter 2009, 26(3): 3).

6. **a**   When the attending physician does not confirm the results of the radiology report for inpatient coding, query the attending physician regarding the clinical significance of the findings and request that appropriate documentation be provided (*Coding Clinic* 2nd Quarter 2002, 17). This is an example of a circumstance where the chronic condition must be verified. All secondary conditions must meet the UHDDS definitions; it is not clear if COPD does (*Coding Clinic* 1st Quarter 2004, 21(1): 20–21).

7. **d**   Coding strictly from the pathology report is not appropriate as the coder is assigning a diagnosis without the attending physician's corroboration. It is therefore appropriate to query the physician (*Coding Clinic* 1st Quarter 2004, 2(1): 20–21).

8. **c**   Excisional debridement can be performed in the operating room, the emergency department, or at the bedside. Coders are encouraged to work with the physician and other healthcare providers to ensure that the documentation in the health record is very specific regarding the type of debridement performed. If there is any question as to whether the debridement is excisional or nonexcisional, the provider should be queried for clarification (Schraffenberger 2012, 297).

9. **b**   When a patient is readmitted because a complication has developed following discharge for a treated miscarriage, a code from category 639 is assigned as the principal diagnosis. The 639 code is used because the miscarriage (spontaneous abortion) was dealt with in a prior episode of care (Schraffenberger 2012, 266–267).

10. **d**   The Medicare Conditions of Participation and the Joint Commission require that the medical record is completed no later than 30 days following discharge of the patient (LaTour and Eichenwald Maki, 2010, 215).

11. **a** If an error is corrected, the healthcare provider who made the error should draw a single line through the error, add a note explaining the error, initial and date it, and add the correct information in chronological order (LaTour and Eichenwald Maki 2010, 213). Further, AHIMA principles for health record documentation specify the prior statement as the proper method for correcting an error in the paper-based records in order to maintain a legally sound record This process is based on the ASTM and HL7 standards for error correction. (AHIMA e-HIM Work Group on Maintaining the Legal EHR. 2005).

12. **b** In order to determine if a medical record is complete, it must be reviewed for certain basic reports including the presence of a history and physical, signed progress notes, and a discharge summary if applicable (LaTour and Eichenwald Maki 2010, 213). The incident report should never be filed in the medical record (John 2011, 653); voided prescription pads are not used during a patient hospitalization; personal case notes from mental health providers are kept separate from the official record. While there are a number of documents required for the hospital medical record to be complete, the ones described in option b present the best answer (McWay 2003, 164).

13. **d** Code 414.01 is assigned to show coronary artery disease in a native coronary artery and is used when a patient has coronary artery disease and no history of coronary bypass graft (CABG) surgery (Schraffenberger 2012, 190–192). Code 93458 includes intraprocedural injection(s) for left ventricular/left atrial angiography, imaging supervision, and interpretation when performed (AMA *CPT Professional Edition* 2013, Cardiac Catheterization Guidelines, 500-503).

14. **a** Common reasons for revision joint replacement surgery include mechanical loosening of the prosthesis, dislocation of the prosthetic joint, fracture of the bone around the implant. To classify mechanical reasons for revision joint replacement, ICD-9-CM diagnosis codes 996.40–996.49 are provided. In addition to one of these codes, the patient should also be assigned a code from the V43.60–V43.69 range to identify the joint previously replaced by prosthesis. The note in the Tabular Index directs the coder to add an additional code for the type of bearing surface. Revision of the acetabular component involves removal and exchange of the entire acetabular component, including both the metal shell and the polyethylene, ceramic, or metal modular bearing surface. Common indications for acetabular component revision are wear of the modular bearing surface, aseptic loosening, malposition of the component, or infection (Brown 2012, 458; *Coding Clinic* 1997 3rd Quarter, 14(3): 13).

15. **b** When an admission involves delivery, the principal diagnosis should identify the main circumstance or complication of the delivery. The 650 code cannot be used because there is a complication of pregnancy because the pregnancy is prolonged. The difference between 645.11 and 645.21 is that 645.1x represents more than 40 completed weeks to 42 completed weeks while 645.2x represents gestation of beyond 42 weeks (Schraffenberger 2012, chapter 14; *Coding Clinic* 4th Quarter 2000, 17(4): 43).

16. **b** ICD-10-CM was developed under the leadership of the National Center for Health Statistics (NCHS), a federal agency under the Centers for Disease Control (CDC). Full compliance is expected for claims received for encounters and discharges occurring on or after 10/1/2014 (Brown 2012, 474).

17. **a** Pseudoaneurysm usually occurs at the site of previous vascular surgery or vessel puncture, which occurs secondary to a rent or defect in the vessel. The vessel was intentionally punctured in order to accomplish the procedure. This type of problem should not be assigned to code 998.2, Accidental puncture or laceration during a procedure (*Coding Clinic* 3rd Quarter 2002, 19(3): 24–27).

18. **d**   Patients with acute ischemic heart disease or acute myocardial ischemia does not always indicate an infarction. It is often possible to prevent infarction by means of surgery or the use of thrombolytic agents if the patient is treated promptly. If there is occlusion or thrombosis of the artery without infarction, code 411.81, Acute coronary occlusion without myocardial infarction, is assigned (Brown 2012, 337; *Coding Clinic* 3rd Quarter 1989, 6(3): 4–5).

19. **d**   Nausea, vomiting, and abdominal pain are symptoms of acute cholecystitis. Signs and symptoms that are associated routinely with a disease process should not be assigned as additional codes, unless otherwise instructed by the classification (HHS 2011, Section I, B, 7).

20. **c**   If the findings are outside the normal range and the attending provider has ordered other tests to evaluate the condition or prescribed treatment, it is appropriate to ask the provider whether the abnormal findings should be added. Abnormal findings from laboratory, x-ray, pathologic, and other diagnostic results are not usually coded and reported unless the physician indicates their clinical significance (Brown 2012, 99).

21. **b**   Code 458.2, Iatrogenic hypotension, should be assigned to describe this condition. This code should be assigned when hypotension develops as a result of any type of medical care. Assign code E941.2, Sympathomimetics (adrenergics), to indicate that it is an adverse effect of the drug (*Coding Clinic* 3rd Quarter 2002, 19(3): 12).

22. **b**   A tear in the dura that occurs during spinal surgery is not unusual and is typically repaired intraoperatively when identified. Primary closure of the dural tear is usually accomplished. Dural tears that are not discovered during surgery can result in leakage of cerebrospinal fluid (CSF), leading to CSF headache, caudal displacement of the brain, subdural hematoma, spinal meningitis, pseudomeningocele and/or a dural cutaneous fistula (*Coding Clinic* 4th Quarter 2008, 109–110).

23. **a**   Respiratory failure may be listed as a secondary diagnosis if it occurs after admission, or if it is present on admission, but does not meet the definition of principal diagnosis (Brown 2012, 189–191; *Coding Clinic* 2nd Quarter 2000, 17(2): 22).

24. **b**   Code 481, Pneumococcal pneumonia, is assigned when both conditions exist. Code also 038.2, Pneumococcal septicemia as well as the SIRS (*Coding Clinic* 1st Quarter 1999, 13; HHS 2011, Section I, C, 1, b, 2, a).

25. **b**   Patients who have undergone kidney transplant may still have some form of CKD, because the kidney transplant may not fully restore kidney function. Therefore, the presence of CKD alone does not constitute a transplant complication. Assign the appropriate 585 code for the patient's end-stage renal disease and code V42.0 (HHS 2011, Section I, C, 10, a, 2).

26. **c**   The condition after study that occasioned the admission should be sequenced first even if the plan of treatment was not carried out due to unforeseen circumstances (HHS 2011, Section II.F).

27. **c**   Incorporating internal and external auditing into the coding compliance plan has proven to be the best strategy. Internal auditing enables managers to see firsthand where their units' strengths and weaknesses lie. External auditing provides an unbiased view of a department's performance. Together, internal and external audits help coding managers build effective education plans for their units (Castro and Layman 2011, 43).

28. **d** Before any unlisted code is assigned, the coding professional should review HCPCS Level II (national) codes to confirm that CMS has not developed a specific code for the procedure or service in question. CPT Category III codes, which are developed specifically for reporting new technology, should also be reviewed. CPT guidelines support the use of a Category III code instead of a Category I unlisted code (Smith 2013, 24).

29. **a** CT colonography uses CT scanning to obtain an interior view of the colon (the large intestine) that is otherwise only seen with a more invasive procedure where an endoscope is inserted into the rectum (Kuehn 2012, 159). *Note:* Code 0066T has been deleted and the coder is instructed to use 74263. Computed tomographic (CT) colonography, screening, including image post-processing (AMA *CPT Professional Edition* 2013, 384).

30. **c** 11602: Excision malignant lesion of trunk . . . excised diameter 1.1 cm to 2.0 cm. The size of the lesion plus the margins are included in coding the excision. Excised diameter: 1.0 cm + 0.2 cm + 0.2 cm = 1.4 cm (Smith 2013, 61).

31. **c** Assign code 80.59, Other destruction of intervertebral disc, for the procedure performed. IDET involves only the disc not the nerve root. IDET is done with thermal energy (heat) directed into the outer disc wall (annulus) and inner disc contents (nucleus) via a heating coil, decreasing the pressure inside the disc. Code 04.2, Destruction of cranial and peripheral nerves, would not be the correct code assignment, because it relates to the peripheral nerves (*Coding Clinic* 3rd Quarter 2002, 10).

32. **c** For tubal ligation, which may be performed by ligation, transaction, or other occlusion of the fallopian tubes, the coder should refer to codes 58600–58615 for abdominal or vaginal approaches. For laparoscopic tubal ligation with the use of Falope rings, code 58671 is assigned (Kuehn 2012, 184).

33. **c** Codes (52234–52240) should only be reported once, regardless of the number of tumors removed. Only one of the three codes may be reported per session. Select the code based on the largest tumor. Code 52240 is used when one or more of the tumors are larger than 5.0 cm (*CPT Assistant* August 2009, 19(8):6).

34. **c** A variety of substances can be injected into the submucosal space of the digestive tract through a sheathed needle-tipped catheter inserted through an endoscope (*CPT Assistant* May 2005, 15(5): 3–6).

35. **c** The endometrial biopsy (58110) is an add-on code and there are specific directions in the CPT book to use this code in conjunction with the code for the colposcopy; (*CPT Changes 2006—An Insider's View; CPT Assistant* June 2006, 16–17).

36. **c** CPT code 52204 is reported only once, irrespective of how many biopsy specimens are obtained and how the specimens are sent for pathologic examination (*CPT Assistant* August 2009, 19(8):6).

37. **d** The operative report should be reviewed for the body part involved with the lesion. The total size of the excised area, including margins, is needed for accurate coding. The pathology report typically provides the specimen size rather than the lesion or excised size. Because the specimen tends to shrink, this is not an accurate measurement according to the intent of the code assignment (Smith 2013, 60-63).

38. **b** The size of the joint is a key determination because arthrocentesis codes are based on whether the joint is small, intermediate, or major (AMA 2013, 95).

39. **c** The blood gas values of pO$_2$ of 58, pCO$_2$ of 55, pH of 7.32 reflect respiratory failure and the patient was treated in ICU with intubation and mechanical ventilation DRG: 0207, RESPIRATORY SYSTEM DIAGNOSIS W VENTILATOR SUPPORT 96+ HOURS. The addition of procedure codes for the intubation and ventilation would move this to MS-DRG 207. The acute exacerbation of COPD with blood gas values of pO$_2$ of 58, pCO$_2$ of 55, pH of 7.32 reflects possible respiratory failure. The patient was treated with intubation and mechanical ventilation for more than 96 hours. MS-DRG 0207 is a correct reflection of the patient's severity illness and appropriate reimbursement resulting based on the documentation when compared to the MS-DRG associated with acute exacerbation of COPD (491.21), which is MS-DRG 192 (weight = 0.7081) (Medicare Grouper Version: 29-10/11).

40. **b** MS-DRG 291 (weight = 01.5010) for congestive heart failure with stage III pressure ulcer would optimize the MS-DRG. MS-DRG 293 (weight = 0. 6756) is assigned for congestive heart failure alone, with atrial fibrillation, with blood loss anemia, and with coronary artery disease all remain the same (Medicare Grouper Version 29-10/11).

41. **d** MS-DRG 264 (weight = 02.5580) for myocardial infarction with transbronchial lung biopsy would result in the highest reimbursement. MS-DRG 282 (weight = 0.7856) would be assigned for the myocardial infarction alone, and with insertion central venous catheter. MS-DRG 282 (weight = 0.7856) would be assigned for myocardial infarction with mechanical ventilator (Medicare Grouper Version 29-10/11).

42. **d** The principal diagnosis should be the condition established after study that was responsible for the patient's admission. If the patient was admitted with a condition that resulted in the performance of a cesarean procedure, which condition should be selected as the principal diagnosis? If the reason for the admission/encounter was unrelated to the condition resulting in the cesarean delivery, the condition related to the reason for the admission/encounter should be selected as the principal diagnosis, even if a cesarean were performed (HHS 2011, Section I, C, 11, b, 4).

43. **d** This patient was previously treated for the spontaneous abortion but the presence of the products of conception denotes that the abortion was not completed during the prior episode of care. Because of this and the fact that she now has sepsis, she is coded as having an incomplete spontaneous abortion with sepsis (Brown 2012, 294).

44. **a** MS-DRG 280 (weight = 01.7901) for myocardial infarction with respiratory failure would change the MS-DRG. MS-DRG 282 (weight = 0.7856) would be assigned for myocardial infarction alone, with atrial fibrillation, with hypertension, and with history of myocardial infarction (Medicare Grouper Version 29-10/11).

45. **c** Pneumonia, diabetes, hypertension should be coded. The migraine headaches are a past condition and would not be coded as per the reporting guidelines for the UHDDS for "other conditions" (HHS 2011, Section III).

46. **b** Pressure ulcer, diabetic neuropathy and diabetic retinopathy, and blindness should be coded. Diabetes and related conditions are chronic conditions that ordinarily should be coded and the patient required nursing care because of her blindness (Brown 2012, 32).

47. **b** The hernia is an incidental finding. The condition does not meet the UHDDS criteria of an "other" condition (Brown 2012, 33).

48. **d**   Query the physician regarding whether a diagnosis should be assigned or not. It is not within the coder's scope of practice to diagnose a condition (Brown 2012, 33).

49. **c**   Payment status indicators that are assigned to an APC and indicate APC payment are G, H, K, P, R, S, T, U, X, and V. Status indicator N denotes that there is no specific payment for that APC because the procedure payment is included in another APC. There may be multiple APCs with the same or different payment status indicator per claim. In this case, all APCs impact payment except the one with status indicator N (Casto and Layman 2011, 185).

50. **d**   Multiple surgical procedures with payment status indicator T performed during the same operative session are discounted. The highest-weighted status T procedure is fully reimbursed. All other procedures with payment status indicator T are reimbursed at 50%. In this case there is only one status T procedure and it is paid 100% (Casto and Layman 2011, 183).

51. **a**   Multiple surgical procedures with payment status indicator T performed during the same operative session are discounted. The highest-weighted procedure is fully reimbursed. All other procedures with payment status indicator T are reimbursed at 50%. Because of this, if another T procedure were codes, it would be reimbursed at 50% (Casto and Layman 2011, 183).

52. **d**   The codes are differentiated according to the route of administration. For Medicare cases, a Level II HCPCS code (J series) is reported with the identification of the specific substance or drug; for non-Medicare cases, code 99070 may be reported. In this case, use both 96372 and J056 (Smith 2012, 255-259). *Note:* HCPCS codes are used in the multiple choice questions but are not assigned when coding the cases on the CCS exam. Refer to the Procedures for Coding Medical Record Cases for the CCS Examination in the Introduction of this book.

53. **d**   Several tools and references are used to support the reimbursement process including the fee schedule and the current National Correct Coding Initiatives edits. Other valuable resources are Medicare's Carrier Manual, Medicare's National Coverage Determinations Manual, and local coverage determinations (LCDs) (Hazelwood and Venable 2011, 292).

54. **a**   The UHDDS item 11-b defines *other diagnoses* as "all conditions that coexist at the time of admission, that develop subsequently or that affect the treatment received or the length of stay" (HHS 2011, Section III).

55. **a**   Assign a diagnostic code for mitral regurgitation. If the diagnostic test has been interpreted by a physician the coder can assign a diagnosis (Brown 2012, 33).

56. **a**   Assign codes for malignant melanoma of forearm, hypertension. Code chronic conditions if they affect the patient's treatment. The hypertension was being treated with a current medication and for this reason the hypertension is coded (Brown 2012, 32).

57. **d**   Do not assign a code for this condition because this is a frequent condition in the elderly, is asymptomatic, and there is no documentation of treating the condition so it should not be coded (Brown 2012, 33).

58. **d**   Assign a code for the chief complaint as the reason for the visit in the absence of a diagnosis or defined problem, the chief compliant should be coded as the reason for the visit (Brown 2012, 34).

59. **b**   The OCE has four basic functions: editing the data on the claims for accuracy, specifying the action the FI should taken when specific edits occur, assigning APCs to the claim (for hospital outpatient services), and determining payment-related conditions that require direct reference to HCPCS codes or modifiers. Routine edits for age and sex are done on all claims (Smith 2013, 266).

60. **c**   The *case mix* is defined as a methods of grouping patients. MS-DRGs are often used to determine case mix in hospitals. The *case-mix index* is the average MS-DRG weight based on the specific patient group and is determined by multiplying the DRG weights by the number of patients and then divided by the total number of patients: $30 + 20 + 10 = 60 / 30 = 2.0$ (LaTour and Eichenwald Maki 2011, 436).

61. **a**   MS-DRG 195 (weight $= 3.0$) Simple pneumonia and pleurisy age >17 w/CC results in higher reimbursement than MS-DRG 193 (weight $= 2.0$) Simple pneumonia without MCC or CC. Note that these are not actual weights for these DRGs.

62. **d**   In the paper chart, a line can be drawn through an erroneous entry, initialed, and the correction made along the margin. In an electronic record, the correction may be placed in the wrong sequence, which may adversely impact patient care (Johns 2011, 183).

63. **c**   For reporting purposes the definition for *other diagnoses* is interpreted as additional conditions that affect patient care in terms of requiring: clinical evaluation; or therapeutic treatment; or diagnostic procedures; or extended length of hospital stay; or increased nursing care or monitoring (HHS 2011, Section III).

64. **d**   The use or application of the data and the purpose for the collection of the data is key to understanding its quality (LaTour and Eichenwald Maki 2010, 117).

65. **d**   Information is used for many purposes and therefore lack of data quality affects many areas (LaTour and Eichenwald Maki 2010, 117).

66. **c**   Unprocessed data are not useful for decision making and for this reason processing data creates information that is useful (LaTour and Eichenwald Maki 2010, 112).

67. **c**   The goal of information management is to support decision making (LaTour and Eichenwald Maki 2010, 114).

68. **c**   Data mining is associated with data warehouses. *Data mining* is a process that identifies patterns and relationships by searching through large amounts of data. Because data warehouses contain large amounts of data, data mining processes are frequently used to systematically analyze these data. In healthcare, data mining is used to identify methods for cutting healthcare costs, suggest more appropriate medical treatments, and predict medical outcomes (Johns 2011, 910).

69. **c**   *DRG groupers* are software programs that help coders determine the appropriate diagnosis-related group (DRG) assignment based on the logic of the system for hospital inpatients. APC groupers are software programs that help coders determine the appropriate ambulatory payment classification for an outpatient encounter (Johns 2011, 449).

70. **a**   An *information system* (IS) consists of data, people, and work processes and a combination of hardware (machines and media), software (computer programs), and communication technology (computer networks) known as information technology (IT) (Johns 2011, 876).

71. **d** Health information exchanges (HIEs) are created to connect providers, patients, payers, and other parties through telecommunication and computer networks, thus enabling data transfer as needed (Johns 2011, 910).

72. **c** Cryptography is a field that develops methods to ensure data security. A digital signature scheme is a public key that ensures a document is authentic (Johns 2011, 922–923).

73. **d** There are many types of malware including viruses, spyware and backdoor. A bus topology is a method of data flow through a network where each computer is connected to a common backbone through a connector. (Johns 2011, 915, 927).

74. **c** By definition, clinical information systems are designed to support patient care but may also be used for quality improvement, peer review, or research, all of which ultimately contribute to better patient care (Johns 2011, 946).

75. **c** Reviewing the history and physical of a coworker when not part of assigned work is not ethical because the review is not part of designated work. This violates the ethical principal of acting with integrity and behaving in a trustworthy manner (AHIMA 2011).

76. **a** The HIM professional must know the retention statutes and retention periods in his or her state of employment (LaTour and Eichenwald Maki 2011, 282).

77. **b** The role of the *risk manager* is to collect and analyze information on actual losses and potential risks and to design systems that lessen potential losses in the future. An incident report is a structured tool used to collect data and information about any event not consistent with routine operational procedures (Johns 2011, 653).

78. **a** *Coding compliance policies* serve as a guide to performing coding and billing functions and provide documentation of the organizations' intent to correctly report services. The policies should include facility-specific documentation requirements, payer regulations and policies, and contractual arrangements for coding consultants and outsourcing services. This information may be covered in payer/provider contracts or found in Medicare and Medicaid manuals and bulletins (AHIMA 2008, 83–88).

79. **b** As of August 17, 2000, HHS published the final regulations for electronic transactions and coding standards as established under HIPAA in the *Federal Register* (65 FR 50312; Schraffenberger 2012, xiv).

80. **d** When a symptom is followed by contrasting or comparative diagnoses, the symptom is sequenced first. All the contrasting or comparative diagnosis should be coded as additional diagnoses (HHS 2011, Section II, E).

81. **b** *External cause of injury codes* are used to provide information about how an injury occurred, the intent (intentional or unintentional), provide information about where the injury occurred, and the status of the person at the time the injury occurred. In the case of a person who seeks care for an injury or other health condition that resulted from an activity, or when an activity contributed to the injury or health condition, activity codes are used to describe the activity (Brown 2012, 406–409).

82. **a, b, e, f**   These elements are used to determine the MS-DRG) MS-DRG assignment goes through four steps: Pre-MDC assignments, MDC determination, Medical/surgical determination, and refinement. These steps are based on surgical procedure codes, diagnosis codes, complications and/or comorbidities, and discharge disposition and other patients characteristics (Schraffenberger 2012, 473).

83. **a, b, c, d, f**   These elements are used to determine the MS-DRG) hospital payment calculation is based on MS-DRG assignment (therefore the MS-DRG weight), establishment of initial payment rate (therefore hospital base rate), add-on for disproportionate share hospitals, add-on for indirect medical education (for teaching hospitals), add-on for high-cost outliers, and add-on for new medical service and technology (Schraffenberger 2012, 472).

84. **b, c, e**   These activities are part of the claims review required by QIOs) These responsibilities are delineated in the Center for Medicare and Medicaid website, as well (CMS 2012, https://www.cms.gov/QualityImprovementOrgs).

85. **b, e, f**   *Medical necessity* is "a service or supply provided for the diagnosis, treatment, cure or relief of health conditions, illness, injury, or disease." These services must be necessary and appropriate and within generally accepted standards of medical care. They must not be provided simply for convenience (Casto and Layman 2010, 99).

86. **a, d**   Code 51.41 is assigned in this case in addition to 51.22 since this was an exploration with removal of stones (*Coding Clinic* 1st Quarter 1996, 12–13).

87. **d, h**   The same reasons presented above apply in this scenario as well, except that the approaches are different. (Brown 2012, 206–207).

88. **b, d, h**   Intraoperative cholangiogram is a valid OR procedure and should be coded (*Coding Clinic* 1st Quarter 1996, 12–13). Also, the incidental appendectomy is coded (*Coding Clinic* 4th Quarter 1996, 65).

89. **a, c, e, f**   If the instruction "omit code" is found next to the code in the Alphabetic Index, this notes the code should not be assigned (Brown 2012, 68).

EXAM 1—PATIENT 1

PDX	233.0	Carcinoma in situ of breast
PP1	19301–RT	Mastectomy, partial (eg, lumpectomy, tylectomy, quadrantectomy, segmentectomy)
PR2	38525	Biopsy or excision of lymph node(s); open, deep axillary node(s)
PR3	38792	Injection procedure; radioactive tracer for identification of sentinel node

Notes on Outpatient 1

233.0   This is an example of carcinoma in-situ of the breast. By looking up the morphologic type of carcinoma, in situ, intraductal of specified site in the Alphabetic Index, the coder is directed to "see neoplasm, by site, in situ" (Brown 2012, 377).

19301–RT   The patient underwent a lumpectomy. The modifier –RT is also important because the breast is a paired organ (*CPT Assistant* Feb. 2007, 4; Dec. 2007, 8; Sept. 2008, 5, March 2010, 10).

38525   Sentinel lymph node dissection was undertaken (*CPT Assistant* May 1998, 10; July 1999, 7; Oct. 2005, 23; Dec. 2007, 8; Sept. 2008, 5).

38792   The injection of radioactive tracer to visualize the sentinel node in the OR may be reported separately with code 38792 (*CPT Assistant* July 1999, 7, 12; *CPT Changes: An Insider's View* 2008, 2012).

EXAM 1—PATIENT 2

PDX	381.10	Chronic serous otitis media, simple or unspecified
DX2	473.9	Unspecified sinusitis (chronic)
DX3	474.12	Hypertrophy of adenoids alone
PP1	69436–50	Tympanostomy (requiring insertion of ventilating tube), general anesthesia (bilateral)
PR2	42831	Adenoidectomy, primary; age 12 or older (Patient is 35 years old.)

Notes on Outpatient 2

381.10   The patient has chronic serous otitis media (the specific documentation of "serous otitis media" is found in the postoperative diagnosis in the operative report) (Schraffenberger 2012, 165).

473.9,
474.12   The patient also has chronic sinusitis and adenoid hypertrophy (Brown 2012, chapter 15).

69436–50   The patient had a bilateral tympanostomy. Modifier –50 is used to identify the bilateral procedure (rather than listing the procedure code twice) (AMA *CPT Professional Edition* 2013, Modifier Section, inside front cover).

42831   The patient also had adenoidectomy. This code is affected by age (AMA *CPT Professional Edition* 2013, 238).

EXAM 1 — PATIENT 3

PDX	371.23	Bullous keratopathy
DX2	379.31	Aphakia
DX3	365.10	Open-angle glaucoma, unspecified
DX4	364.10	Chronic iridocyclitis, unspecified
DX5	413.9	Other and unspecified angina pectoris
DX6	496	Chronic airway obstruction (COPD)
PP1	65750–LT	Keratoplasty (corneal transplant); penetrating (in aphakia)
PR2	66985–LT	Insertion of intraocular lens prosthesis (secondary implant), not associated with concurrent cataract removal
PR3	67010–LT	Removal of vitreous, anterior approach (open sky technique or limbal incision); subtotal removal with mechanical vitrectomy

Notes on Outpatient 3

371.23, 379.31, 365.10, 364.10	The conditions specified in the record should be coded (Brown 2012, 169–173).
413.9	Angina should be coded as it meets the UHDDS definition of another diagnosis (Brown 2012, 338).
496	COPD should be coded as it meets the UHDDS definition of another diagnosis (Brown 2012, 186–188).
Note:	History of prostate cancer is not coded because it does not have an effect on the current encounter (Brown 2012, 90).
Note:	The –LT modifier denoting the left eye is used on all of the procedure codes:

65750–LT   *CPT Assistant* Oct. 2002, 8; April 2009, 5; Dec. 2009, 13

66985–LT   *CPT Assistant* Sept. 2005, 12; Sept. 2009, 5

67010–LT   *CPT Assistant* Fall 1992, 4

EXAM 1—PATIENT 4

PDX	872.01	Open wound of ear, auricle
PP1	12011	Simple repair of superficial wounds of face, ears, eyelids, nose, lips and/or mucous membranes; 2.5 cm or less (2 cm laceration specified in the physical examination)
PR2	99283–25	E/M code based on mapping scenario provided (40 total points*)

Notes on Outpatient 4

872.01   The laceration is of the external ear, of the auricle.

12011   A simple repair of the ear was done of less than 2.5 cm (*CPT Assistant* Feb. 2000, 10; May 2000, 8; Jan. 2002, 10; Feb. 2008, 8). The repair is of the skin and therefore no modifier for the left side is assigned.

99283–25   The coder will need to calculate the E/M code for the outpatient visit. *According to the mapping scenario; meds given are = 1 = 5 points, the history is problem focused = 10 points, the exam is problem focused = 10 points, the number of tests = 0 = 5 points, supplies = 2 suture kits = 10 points. This equals 40 points.

         In Section IV of the Official Coding Guidelines, guidance is given related to how to sequence the diagnostic codes. Generally, if there is surgery, the reason for the surgery is sequenced first as it is the reason for the encounter. The related procedure or E/M code is sequenced to match the diagnosis. In this case, the patient came to the ED to repair her ear laceration. This is the reason that the sutures were sequenced first.

EXAM 1—PATIENT 5

PDX	812.21	Fracture of humerus, shaft of humerus
DX2	305.1	Tobacco use disorder
PP1	24505–LT	Closed treatment of humeral shaft fracture; with manipulation, with or without skeletal traction
PR2	99284–25	E/M code based on mapping scenario provided (50 total points*)

Notes on Outpatient 5

812.21   The patient has sustained a fracture of the humerus (Brown 2012, 412–417).

305.1   The patient received tobacco cessation counseling and instructions to see her primary care physician (Schraffenberger 2012, 147).

24505–LT   In CPT, reduction is termed treatment of fracture with manipulation.

99284–25   Calculate the evaluation and management code for the outpatient visit. *According to the mapping scenario; meds given are = 2 = 5 points, the history is problem focused = 10 points, the exam is extended problem focused = 15 points, the number of tests = 5 = 15 points, supplies = 1 fracture tray = 5 points. Total is 50 points.

EXAM 1 — PATIENT 6

PDX	414.01	Coronary atherosclerosis of native coronary artery
PP1	93460	Catheter placement in coronary artery(s) for coronary angiography, including intraprocedural injection(s) for coronary angiography, imaging supervision and interpretation; with right and left heart catheterization including intraprocedural injection(s) for left ventriculography, when performed.
PR2	93567	Injection procedure during cardiac catheterization including imaging supervision, interpretation, and report; for supravalvular aortography (List separately in addition to code to code for primary procedure.)

Notes on Outpatient 6

414.01   The patient has arteriosclerotic heart disease with no history of cardiac bypass (Schraffenberger 2012, 190–192).

93460   Catheter placement in coronary artery(s) for coronary angiography, including intraprocedural injection(s) for coronary angiography, imaging supervision and interpretation; with right and left heart catheterization including intraprocedural injection(s) for left ventriculography, when performed (Kuehn 2012, 261–262).

+93567   Injection procedure during cardiac catheterization including imaging supervision, interpretation, and report; for supravalvular aortography. (List separately in addition to code to code for primary procedure.)

EXAM 1 — PATIENT 7

PDX	197.7	Secondary malignant neoplasm of liver
DX2	162.5	Malignant neoplasm of lung, lower lobe
PP1	10022	Fine needle aspiration; with imaging guidance
PR2	76942	Ultrasonic guidance for needle placement (e.g., biopsy, aspiration, injection, localization device), imaging supervision and interpretation

Notes on Outpatient 7

197.7   The patient is being seen because of the metastatic cancer of the liver (Brown 2012, 384–386).

162.5   The patient's primary site is the right lower lobe of the lung (Brown 2012, 380–384).

10022   The patient undergoes a fine needle aspiration with imaging guidance (CPT Assistant, Nov. 2002, 1; June 2007, 10).

76942   The ultrasound guidance is also coded (CPT Assistant Fall 1993, 12; Fall 1994, 2; May 1996, 3; June 1997, 5; Oct. 2001, 2; May 2004, 7; Dec. 2004, 12; April 2005, 15–16; Aug. 2008, 7; March 2009, 8).

EXAM 1—PATIENT 8

PDX	820.21	Fracture of neck of femur, intertrochanteric section
DX2	997.5	Urinary complications
DX3	788.20	Retention of urinary, unspecified
DX4	428.0	Congestive heart failure, unspecified
DX5	562.10	Diverticulosis of colon (without mention of hemorrhage)
DX6	424.0	Mitral valve disorders
DX7	414.01	Coronary atherosclerosis of native coronary artery
DX8	V12.71	History of peptic ulcer disease
DX9	715.90	Osteoarthritis, unspecified
DX10	290.0	Senile dementia, uncomplicated
PP1	79.35	Open reduction with internal fixation of femur

Notes on Inpatient 8

820.21   Radiology report denotes intertrochanteric fracture (Brown 2012, 412–414).

997.5   Patient had postoperative urinary retention as documented in the 12/1 progress note. The 997 category directs coders to use an additional code to identify the specific complication in addition to 997 (*Coding Clinic* 2nd Quarter, 1998).

788.20   Patient had postoperative urinary retention as documented in the 12/1 progress note. The 997 category directs coders to use an additional code to identify the specific complication in addition to 997(*Coding Clinic* 2nd Quarter, 1998).

428.0   Congestive heart failure (Brown 2012, 339–340).

562.10   The patient has diverticulosis (Brown 2012, 205)

424.0   Aortic valve disorder (Brown 2012, 330–332).

414.01   Arteriosclerotic heart disease (Brown 2012, 330–332).

V12.71   The patient has a history of peptic ulcer (Brown 2012, 83).

715.90   The patient has osteoarthritis (Brown 2012, 253).

290.00   The patient has senile dementia (Brown 2012, 135–137).

79.35   The patient underwent open reduction with internal fixation (Brown 2012, 410–411).

Note: Per the Procedures for Coding Medical Record Cases for the CCS Examination, "Do not code 57.94 (Foley catheter)."

Points of Interest on Inpatient 8

1. This case provides an example of postoperative urinary retention, which is a commonly missed complication.

2. You must review the radiology report to determine where the fracture is. This is frequently the case with coding actual records.

EXAM 1—PATIENT 9

PDX	663.31	Delivery complicated by nuchal cord without compression
DX2	V27.0	Single liveborn
DX3	648.61	Other cardiovascular diseases in the mother classifiable elsewhere, but complicating pregnancy, childbirth, or the puerperium
DX4	424.0	Mitral valve disorders
PP1	73.6	Episiotomy

Notes on Inpatient 9

663.31 As per the delivery note, this is a delivery with a nuchal cord wrapped around the baby's neck (Brown 2012, 289).

V27.0 Outcome of delivery code (Brown 2012, 270).

648.61, 424.0 These must be coded because they affected the monitoring of the patient and were documented in the medical record. The "use additional code" note at category 648 directs the coder to add another code to identify the condition (Brown 2012, 276–277).

73.6 Episiotomy—the repair of an episiotomy is included in the code (Brown 2012, 282).

Points of Interest on Patient 9

1. In terms of documentation, this case is typical of many delivery charts. Often times, practitioners document the complication of delivery in only one area, such as the delivery note or the operative report. In this case, the baby has a nuchal cord, but it is only mentioned once in the delivery record.

2. This is also an illustration of the three types of codes, at a minimum, that must be on every delivery chart: a diagnostic code from the delivery or pregnancy category, an outcome of birth code (V code), and a procedure code.

EXAM 1—PATIENT 10

PDX	482.83	Pneumonia due to other gram-negative bacteria
DX2	250.52	Diabetes with ophthalmic manifestations, type II or unspecified type, uncontrolled
DX3	362.01	Background diabetic retinopathy
DX4	401.9	Essential hypertension, unspecified
DX5	V09.2	Infection with microorganisms resistant to macrolides
DX6	715.36	Osteoarthritis, localized, knees
DX7	424.1	Aortic valve disorders
DX8	V58.67	Long-term (current) use of insulin

Notes on Inpatient 10

482.83   Gram-negative pneumonia documented on the H & P and 2/2 progress note (*Coding Clinic* 3rd Quarter, 1988).

250.52   Noninsulin-dependent diabetes mellitus (insulin requiring) used because the H & P states "Diabetes mellitus–uncontrolled" 1/31 progress note addresses treatment plan for diabetes out of control. Orders of 1/31 and 2/1 reflect treatment. The blood glucose record reflects high blood sugar (*Coding Clinic* 4th Quarter 1997; *Coding Clinic* 2nd Quarter 1997; *Coding Clinic* 2nd Quarter 2002; *Coding Clinic* 3rd Quarter 2002).

362.01   Retinopathy is documented on the discharge summary (Brown 2012, 125).

401.9   Documented on the H & P and discharge summary. The patient is on HCTZ for this condition (Brown 2012, 346–350).

V09.2   Reported because the resistant organism is documented in the discharge summary and laboratory reports. Furthermore, the patient tried erythromycin and needed to be changed to another antibiotic (Brown 2012, 113).

715.36   Documented in the D/C summary, H & P, and the orders (Brown 2012, 253–254).

424.1   Documented in the D/C summary, H & P, and the orders (Brown 2012, 330–332).

V58.67   The patient has been on insulin long term (Brown 2012, 122).

Points of Interest on Inpatient 10

1. The patient has pneumonia and documentation needs to have the organism causing the pneumonia specified in the medical record in areas other than just the sputum culture.

2. The patient also has uncontrolled diabetes as evidenced by the labile blood sugar and the documentation in the record.

3. Coders should only use the V codes denoting resistance when the resistance is documented by the physician(s) involved (Brown 2012, 113).

EXAM 1—PATIENT 11

PDX	162.5	Malignant neoplasm of lung, lower lobe
DX2	997.1	Cardiac complications (Intraoperative myocardial infarction [MI])
DX3	410.71	Acute myocardial infarction, subendocardial infarction
DX4	401.9	Essential hypertension, unspecified
DX5	458.29	Iatrogenic hypotension
DX6	496	Chronic airway obstruction, not elsewhere classified (COPD)
DX7	721.3	Lumbosacral spondylosis without myelopathy
DX8	438.21	Hemiplegia affecting dominant side
DX9	V15.82	History of tobacco use
DX10	V15.3	History of radiation therapy
PP1	32.59	Pneumonectomy

Notes on Inpatient 11

162.5	Recurrent lung cancer is documented in the H & P, discharge summary, and operative report (Brown 2012, 380–386).
997.1	(Brown 2012, 460–461).
410.71	Postoperative/intraoperative myocardial infarction is documented in the progress notes (Brown 2012, 333–335).
401.9	Hypertension documented in the H & P and the D/C summary (Brown 2012, 346–349).
458.29	This is the precipitating factor causing the MI (Brown 2012, 352).
32.59	Pneumonectomy is documented in the operative report.
496, 721.3, 438.21	Should be coded because they are documented in the medical record and are relevant to the admission (HHS 2011, Section III, 89; Brown 2011, chapters 15, 19, 24).
V15.82	History of tobacco use (HHS 2011, Section I, c, 18, d, 4).
V45.76	Partial removal of the lung (HHS 2011, Section I, c, 18, d, 3).
32.59	Removal of the lung is noted in the operative record (Brown 2012, 89–90).

Point of Interest on Inpatient 11

1. This case allows the coder to practice coding an intraoperative complication. Further, the coder needs to differentiate if the myocardial infarction caused the hypotension or if the hypotension caused the myocardial infarction. In this case, the intraoperative hypotension occurred, which resulted in an MI. This case illustrates that problem. This is a clinical scenario about which coders have little education.

EXAM 1 — PATIENT 12

PDX	410.41	Acute myocardial infarction of other inferior wall
DX2	426.0	Atrioventricular block, complete
DX3	578.0	Hematemesis
DX4	285.1	Acute posthemorrhagic anemia
DX5	272.4	Hyperlipidemia
DX6	414.01	Coronary atherosclerosis of native artery
DX7	787.01	Nausea with vomiting
DX8	E938.4	Adverse effect of other and unspecified general anesthetics
DX9	V15.82	History of tobacco use
PP1	36.11	Aortocoronary bypass of one coronary artery
PR2	36.06	Insertion of non-drug-eluting coronary artery stent(s)
PR3	37.22	Left heart cardiac catheterization
PR4	88.55	Coronary arteriography using a single catheter
PR5	88.53	Angiocardiography of left heart structures
PR6	45.13	Other endoscopy of small intestine (EGD)
PR7	00.66	PTCA
PR8	00.45	Insertion of one vascular stent
PR9	00.40	Procedure on single vessel
PR10	39.61	Extracorporeal circulation auxiliary to open heart surgery

Notes on Inpatient 12

410.41   Acute inferior MI is documented on the 4/20 EKG. This is also evident from the laboratory reports because the CK-MB is elevated (Brown 2012, 333–335).

426.0   Complete heart block is documented on the discharge summary, the H & P, and the EKG (Brown 2012, chapter 24).

578.0   Code the hematemesis because no cause has been found (Brown 2012, 201–202).

285.1   Following the upper gastrointestinal bleeding, the patient experienced acute blood loss anemia (Brown 2011, 152).

272.4   Hyperlipidemia is documented on the H & P and summary (Brown 2012, chapter 11).

414.01   Patient is found to have arteriosclerotic heart disease. Code the native artery (fifth digit 1) because the patient has never undergone bypass surgery prior to this admission. Therefore, assume the ASHD is of the native artery (Brown 2012, 337).

787.01   Nausea and vomiting is the adverse effect of a drug (E938.4) (Brown 2012, 445).

E938.4   Adverse effect of anesthesia (Brown 2012, 445).

V15.82   History of tobacco use (Brown 2012, 89–90).

36.11	CABG ×2 on same artery *Coding Clinic* 4th Quarter 1989, 3–5)
36.06	Insertion non-drug-eluting stents (Brown 2012, 361–362).
37.22	Left heart catheterizations (Brown 2012, 355).
88.55	Angiography using a single catheter (Brown 2012, 356).
88.53	Ventriculography (Brown 2012, 356).
45.13	EGD (Brown 2012, chapter 16).
00.66	PTCA (Brown 2012, 361–362).
00.45	Insertion of one vascular stent (Brown 2012, 361–362).
00.40	Procedure on a single vessel (Brown 2012, 361–362).
39.61	Extracorporeal (Brown 2012, 373).

Points of Interest on Patient 12

1. The coder must code the site of the myocardial infarction to obtain the correct fourth digit. Look at the EKG to determine the site of acute inferior myocardial infarction. Keep in mind the coding guideline related to ST elevation myocardial infarction (STEMI) and non-ST elevation myocardial infarction (NSTEMI) (HHS 2011, Section I, 7, e, 1).

2. This case also requires a code for the upper gastrointestinal hemorrhage because there is no specified cause.

3. Recognize nausea and vomiting is an adverse effect of anesthesia.

4. The CABG and the heart catheterization provide practice in this area. Remember stents, if they are placed, by coding with an additional code when coding PTCAs. Also code the angiography and ventriculography, if done. To correctly code these procedures, carefully determine how many catheters are used during the angiography in order to code them appropriately. Note: The heart catheterization and insertion of stent took place on a different date.

5. If extracorporeal circulation is used, code this as directed by the *ICD-9-CM* codebook notation. Cardioplegia would not be coded because this is included in the coronary artery bypass code.

6. Per the Procedures for Coding Medical Record Cases for the CCS Examination, the following procedures would *not* be coded: "Code all procedures that fall within the code range 00.01–86.99, but do not code 57.94 (Foley catheter)." Because of this direction, do not code 99.10 for the TPA. (For Procedures for Coding Medical Record Cases for the CCS Examination, refer to this book's Introduction.)

Practice Exam 2

1. **a** A miscarriage is a spontaneous abortion. If the readmission is for the purpose of dealing with retained products of conception, a code from the 634–637 is assigned along with the fifth digit 1 to indicate it was incomplete (Brown 2012, 294).

2. **a** Recurring mood changes that result in periods of severe depression alternating with extreme elation that are beyond the normal range of mood swings are called bipolar or circular disorders (Brown 2012, 137–138).

3. **d** A cesarean section is performed for a variety of reasons, such as cephalopelvic disproportion (CPD), prolapsed cord, fetal distress, and conditions of the mother. Based on the information given in this case, fetal head was measured and then it was decided a cesarean section should be performed. It is likely that the reason for this was CPD; therefore, physician should be queried (Brown 2012, 273; APA 2007; Lovaasen and Schwerdtfeger 2011, 624).

4. **c** With the documented clinical indicators, it would be appropriate to query the physician regarding the possibility of a complication resulting from surgery. When formulating a query, it is unacceptable to lead a provider to document a particular response. The query should not be directing or probing and the provider should not be led to make an assumption (Lovaasen and Schwerdtfeger 2011, 42).

5. **d** According to *Coding Clinic*, if there is evidence of a diagnosis within the medical record and the coder is uncertain whether it is a valid diagnosis because the documentation is incomplete, it is the coders responsibility to query the attending physician to determine if this diagnosis should be included (AHA 2nd Quarter 2000, 17–18).

6. **b** Esophageal varices are often associated with cirrhosis of the liver. In this case, dual coding is required with the underlying condition coded first. For example, esophageal varices with cirrhosis of liver is coded as 571.5 (cirrhosis of liver) + 456.21 (esophageal varices in diseases classified elsewhere) (Brown 2012, 203).

7. **a** An inpatient is a patient who is provided with room, board, and continuous general nursing services in an area of an acute-care facility where patients generally stay at least overnight (Johns 2011, 705; Scott 2009, 3).

8. **d** The patient is being seen in the emergency department, which is a hospital outpatient department. Because of this, all CPT and HCPCS codes should be captured so that the correct reimbursement is obtained (Kirchoff 2009, 33–42).

9. **b** According to AHIMA documentation guidelines, any additional late entry to the record should be labeled as such and these addenda should be added if the physician is queried but the associated documentation to support the code assignment is not present in the original record. In this case, it is an addendum (Johns 2011, 107).

10. **b** The committee that is responsible for ensuring that medical records are complete is the Medical record Committee but it reports to the Medical Executive Committee (LaTour and Eichenwald Maki 2010, 214).

11. **c** There are many areas that accrediting agencies review but timeliness and legibility of medical documents are two of the most important aspects of medical record management (LaTour and Eichenwald Maki 2010, 213).

12. **d** In a nonteaching hospital only the attending physician needs to sign the documents in the medical record but in teaching hospitals, the attending should co-sign after the resident signs the documentation (LaTour and Eichenwald Maki 2010, 213).

13. **a** When the diagnostic statement lists the symptom first, followed by two or more contrasting or comparative conditions, a symptom may be assigned as a principal diagnosis (Brown 2012, 29–30, 97).

14. **c** In this case, there is documentation of the ventilator associated pneumonia (VAP), therefore, code 997.31, Ventilator associated pneumonia, should be assigned. An additional code to identify the organism should also be assigned (041.7, Pseudomonas aeruginosa). No additional codes from categories 480–484 to identify the type of pneumonia are assigned (HHS 2011, Section I, C, 17, f, 3, a).

15. **d** An adverse reaction can occur when a drug was correctly prescribed and administered. In the case of an adverse reaction, the manifestation is coded first (Hematuria) followed by an E code for the medication (Coumadin) (HHS 2011, Section I, C, 17, e, 1).

16. **c** Pleural effusion can be a symptom of CHF, however, in this case, it can be coded because it meets the definition for coding additional diagnosis (it required a diagnostic procedure and it was still unresolved at discharge (HHS 2011, Section III). The sequencing of the two codes would depend on the documentation.

17. **c** This is a confirmed HIV case; therefore, it should be coded first, followed by the additional diagnosis code for all reported HIV-related conditions. Also, the scenario describes a bacterial pneumonia; therefore, code 482.41 is assigned and 484.8 is not used (HHS 2011, Section I, C, 1, a, 1–2).

18. **d** When assigning codes for diabetes and its associated conditions, the code(s) from category 250 must be sequenced before the codes for the associated conditions. Without additional documentation regarding the specific diabetic manifestation related to the heel ulcer, the only code choice for the diabetes is 250.80 (HHS 2011, Section I, C, 3, a, 4).

19. **d** Heart conditions (425.8, 429.0–429.3, 429.8, 429.9) are assigned to a code from category 402 when a causal relationship is stated (due to hypertension) or implied (hypertensive). Use an additional code from category 428 to identify the type of heart failure in those patients with heart failure (HHS 2011, Section I, C, 7, a, 2).

20. **c** The ICD-9-CM Neoplasm table reference at the beginning of the table provides instruction related to sites marked with the * sign. When referencing *neoplasm, knee* in the table, an * is found after *knee* NEC. The instructions direct the coder as follows: *"Sites marked with the sign * should be classified to malignant neoplasm of skin of these sites...."* Follow that path and code to neoplasm, skin, knee, and the correct answer is 173.72, Malignant neoplasm of skin, skin of lower limb, including hip (Brown 2012, chapter 25).

21. **a**   Alphabetic Index for fracture, orbital, roof guides the coder to see fracture, skull, base. After evaluating the selections for the fourth and fifth digit, the correct answer is 801.00, Fracture of base of skull, closed without mention of intracranial injury, unspecified state of consciousness (Brown 2012, 412–414).

22. **d**   Both burns are at the same body part; therefore, only the highest degree burn should be coded (Brown 2012, 434).

23. **b**   An intentional drug overdose is coded as poisoning. Also, in poisoning cases, E codes should be assigned as necessary to completely describe the cause, intent and place of occurrence (HHS 2011, Section I, C, 17, e, 2, b; Brown 2012, 445).

24. **d**   When the drug was correctly prescribed and properly administered, code the reaction plus the appropriate code from the E930–E949 series. If the specific reaction is not documented, it is appropriate to choose code 995.20 (HHS 2011, Section I, C, 17, e, 1).

25. **d**   533.20, 280.0 The patient has an acute peptic ulcer with perforation and hemorrhage. The patient has chronic blood loss anemia due to the hemorrhage. Blood-loss anemia not otherwise specified is coded to 280.0 and in the absence of specific documentation, this code should be assigned. Combination codes are provided for gastric, gastrojejunal, and duodenal ulcers that indicate whether there is associated bleeding, associated perforation, or both (Brown 2012, 152, 203).

26. **a**   Manipulation refers to the attempted reduction or restoration of a dislocated joint or fracture (Smith 2013, 84–85).

27. **c**   When multiple wounds are repaired with the same closure type (for example, simple), lengths of the wounds in the same classification and from all anatomical sites that are grouped together into the same code descriptor should be added together (Smith 2013, 66–69).

28. **d**   A complex repair of a wound goes beyond a layer closure and requires scar revision, debridement, extensive undermining, stents, or retention sutures (Smith 2013, 67).

29. **a**   Codes 65710–65757 are used to describe keratoplasty or corneal transplants. This case does not mention penetrating but anterior lamellar keratoplasty. Therefore, the correct code assignment is 65710, Keratoplasty (corneal transplant), anterior lamellar (*CPT Changes Insider's View* 2009).

30. **c**   Codes 49650–49659 describe procedures related to laparoscopic hernia repairs. Note that 49657 was a new code in 2009 to specifically describe laparoscopic surgical repair of recurrent incisional hernia, incarcerated (including mesh insertion) (Smith 2013, 126–127).

31. **b**   Code 50593, Ablation, renal tumor(s), unilateral, percutaneous, cryotherapy is used for cryoablation of renal tumors (AMA *CPT Professional Edition* 2013, 280).

32. **c**   CPT codes 92928 would be reported for transcatheter stenting of a single coronary vessel (Smith 2013, 235–237).

33. **a**   Surgery is the only treatment and cure for ventral hernias 53.71, is used for laparoscopic repair of diaphragmatic hernia, abdominal approach (*Coding Clinic* 4th Quarter 2008, 165–169).

34. **b** This episode of care occurs in the ER which is an outpatient setting, therefore, a CPT code should be used. CPT code 36831 correctly identifies the thrombectomy procedure (Kirchoff 2009, 203).

35. **d** A myringotomy for insertion of ventilating tubes is a tympanostomy, which is described by codes 69433–69436. Code 69436, Tympanostomy (requiring insertion of ventilating tube), general anesthesia describes the procedure performed. In addition, this procedure was performed bilaterally, therefore, modifier –50 is added (Smith 2013, 163).

36. **d** According to Smith, the documentation needed to properly code removal of skin tags includes diagnosis of skin tags and the number of skin tags removed. These details are provided in the scenario given, therefore, the correct code assignment is 11200, Removal of skin tags, multiple fibrocutaneous tags, any area; up to and including 15 lesions (Smith 2013, 61).

37. **d** The code 31526 is assigned because the patient had a laryngoscopy with an operating microscope. The use of a microscope and whether or not the laryngoscopy was direct are two key issues that must be considered when assigning the CPT code. Codes 31515–31571 are used to identify a direct laryngoscopy. It is inappropriate to use code 69990, Use of operating microscope, in addition to any laryngoscopy code identified as being done with an operating microscope (AMA 2012, 160; Smith 2013, 97).

38. **c** According to the UHDDS definition of the secondary diagnosis, a secondary or additional diagnosis is the diagnosis which receives clinical evaluation, therapeutic treatment, further evaluation, extends length of stay or increases nursing monitoring/care (HHS 2011, Section II).

39. **b** Beginning in fiscal year 2009, CMS designated stage III and IV pressure ulcers as a hospital acquired condition (HAC). If a HAC diagnosis is present at admission (Y), it will continue to be classified as CC or MCC and will impact MS-DRG reimbursement. If a HAC diagnosis is not present at admission (N), it will no longer be classified as CC or MCC and will decrease MS-DRG reimbursement (Garrett 2009, 11).

40. **c** According to the UHDDS definition of the principal diagnosis is "that condition established after study to be chiefly responsible for occasioning the admission of the patient to the hospital for care." In this case, metastatic carcinoma of the brain is responsible for the patient's fall, ataxia and syncope (HHS 2011, Section II).

41. **b** Congestive heart failure includes symptoms such as shortness of breath and pleural effusion. Since these symptoms are the main reason for admission, congestive heart failure is the probable principal diagnosis (Schraffenberger 2012, 192).

42. **a** This is an instance when two diagnoses equally meet the definition of principal diagnosis; therefore, either of the diagnoses may be sequenced as principal diagnosis (HHS 2011, Section II, C).

43. **a** The postoperative complication that is not present at admission. The insurance company may not pay for the services provided to take care of the postoperative complication (Garrett 2009, 11).

44. **d** A condition that pre-exists before admission is considered a comorbidity and because of its presence there will likely be an increase in the patient's length of stay (Schraffenberger 2012, 65).

45. **b** According to the UHDDS a significant procedure is one that is surgical, carries an increased risk, and requires specialized training. Because of this the only answer that is not part of the definition is b (Schraffenberger 2012, 65).

46. **d** UB-04 supports the transition to ICD-10-CM and ICD-10-PCS. The electronic 837 transaction standard and UB-04 accommodate the national provider identifiers, the health plan identifiers, and migration to the ICD-10-CM and PCS coding systems when they are implemented. This is an increased emphasis on clinical codes (Schraffenberger 2012, 65).

47. **d** The principal diagnosis is defined as the condition "established after study to be chiefly responsible for occasioning the admission of the patient to the hospital for care." Selecting the principal diagnosis depends on the circumstances of the admission and why the patient was admitted (Schraffenberger 2012, 66).

48. **d** The outpatient code editor (OCE) performs four basic functions: editing the data on the claim for accuracy, specifying the action the fiscal intermediary should take when specific edits occur, assigning APCs to the claim (for hospital outpatient services) and determining payment-related conditions that require direct reference to HCPCS codes or modifiers. Choice "d" is not one of these functions (Smith 2013, 266).

49. **d** A colonoscopy is the examination of the entire colon, from the rectum to the cecum, that may include the terminal ileum (AMA *CPT Professional Edition* 2013, 257).

50. **b** When a patient presents for outpatient surgery, code the reason for the surgery as the first-listed diagnosis (reason for the encounter) even if the surgery is not performed due to a contraindication (HHS 2011, Section IV, A, 1).

51. **d** Total reimbursement is $3,300 ($2,000 for the procedure with status indicator S + $50 for the procedure with status indicator X + $1,000 for the first procedure with status indicator T + $250 for the second procedure with status indicator T). Use 50% of the reimbursement for the lower reimbursement APC with status indicator T (Casto and Layman 2011, 175–183).

52. **a** Multiple surgical procedures with payment status indicator T performed during the same operative session are discounted. The highest weighted procedure is fully reimbursed and all procedures with payment status indicator T are reimbursed at 50%. Procedure code 10060 is associated with the lower reimbursement APC with status indicator T, therefore, will be paid at 50% (Casto and Layman, 2011, 175–183).

53. **d** Status S procedures are not discounted when multiple procedures are done (Kirchoff 2009, 12).

54. **d** There is a specific code that should be assigned—795.08 (Schraffenberger 2012, 341).

55. **d** Rule-out conditions are not coded in the outpatient setting and the condition qualified in that statement should not be coded as if it existed, rather the preceding signs and symptoms should be coded (Schraffenberger 2012, 344).

56. **a** Tools have been developed to facilitate communication to resolve differences between handwritten and dictated reports or other instances of disparate communication. Sometimes documentation in the health record or on the charge ticket needs to be corrected or verified. Many offices develop a form as a common communication tool for use between a coder and a physician. This form can be as simple or complex as the office sees fit (Kuehn 2012, 360).

57. **c** In order to ensure that outpatient claims were submitted correctly, Medicare Part B claims processing software was developed and is required (Kuehn 2012, 374).

58. **b** Outpatient prospective payment system (OPPS) is used for outpatient hospital services. A hernia repair procedure can be performed in a hospital outpatient setting, therefore, would be paid under the OPPS (Casto and Layman 2011, 4).

59. **b** A payment status indicator establishes how the service is paid in the hospital outpatient prospective payment methodology (Casto and Layman 2011, 175).

60. **a** There is only one MS-DRG per inpatient discharge but there can be one or more APCs per outpatient visit (Casto and Layman 2011, 180). (Also, refer to the Procedures for Coding Medical Record Cases for the CCS Examination in the Introduction of this book for more details.)

61. **c** The correct answer is 45 ($2.0 \times 10 + 1.5 \times 10 + 1.0 \times 10$). Case mix is the sum of relative weights (LaTour and Eichenwald Maki 2010, 436).

62. **a** Compare MS-DRG relative weights for DRG 191, 192, and 193. The lower the relative weight, the lower the payment. DRG 193 has the lowest weight and therefore admitting more patients in this DRG will only lower the CMI; the payment is lowest for DRG 193. DRG 193 has the lowest weight (Johns 2011, 323).

63. **d** If the data are valid, it means the data are correct (Johns 2011, 509).

64. **b** Edits can be in the form of setting parameters of data type for a given field such as numeric or Yes/No. Anything that is entered that is not the correct data type triggers an edit (Johns 2011, 509).

65. **b** Data are considered to be reliable when the values are consistent (Johns 2011, 47).

66. **d** The disease and procedure indices would be used. Such tasks are usually performed more efficiently by avoiding manual abstraction of the records and utilizing reporting capabilities built in various information systems (LaTour and Eichenwald Maki 2010, 331).

67. **d** The procedure index would be used. Such tasks are usually performed more efficiently by avoiding manual abstraction of the records and utilizing reporting capabilities built in various information systems. In addition to this, filtering the data by using the predetermined RBC values for blood transfusion, will sort out the blood transfusion cases and make the ones who did not follow the predetermined criteria easily identifiable (LaTour and Eichenwald Maki 2011, 331).

68. **d** A billing and reimbursement abstracting system tracks assigned diagnosis and procedure codes and identifies which cases to correct (LaTour and Eichenwald Maki 2011, 331).

69. **c** This legislation provides financial rewards to implementation of EHRs (Johns 2011, 151).

70. **c** Interoperability allows systems to address functional requirements established by standards development organizations (Johns 2011, 151).

71. **c** Coding tasks include review of records assigned, completion of abstracting, and evaluation of coding quality but does not include risk analysis for medical record documentation (AHIMA Standards of Ethical Coding 2008).

72. **d** Routine computer backups are a preventive measure and assure data saving at predetermined intervals; therefore, data loss is minimized in the event of "down time" (Johns 2011, 925–927).

73. **d** This question relates to the need-to-know principle. The medical staff member who is not associated with the patient's care does not need to see that patient's record (Johns 2011, 778–779).

74. **a** In this case, health information is being used for payment purposes, which is part of the Privacy Rule related to TPO—Treatment, Payment, and Operations (Johns 2011, 823).

75. **b** Confidentiality requires that we do not communicate information about a patient or the events that take place with that individual without his consent (Johns 2011, 755).

76. **b** Unless there are extenuating circumstances such as the patient not being alive or being incapacitated, the patient is normally the person who provides consent for the release of information (Johns 2011, 755).

77. **c** Bylaws must include a requirement that a history and physical exam must be completed and documented for each patient no more than 30 days before or 24 hours after admission or registration, but prior to surgery or a procedure requiring anesthesia services (Medicare Conditions of Participation, Medical Staff 2003, 485).

78. **a** Choice "b," is more expensive and not done as frequently as the internal audit. Choices "c," and "d," are not key parts of the internal compliance plans (Schraffenberger and Kuehn 2011, 397).

79. **c** Careful discharge planning ensures proper follow-up medical or nursing care after the patient leaves the hospital. This is continuity of care (Johns 2011, 652).

80. **c** Coding audits performed by physician payers may occur but are not part of the coding compliance plan (Davis and LaCour 2007, 156).

81. **b** There are seven elements including written standards of conduct, designation of a chief compliance officer, education, a method to receive complaints, a system to respond to allegations, use of audits, and investigation and remediation of systemic problems, for a compliance program. Development of a penalty fund is not one of the seven elements (LaTour and Eichenwald Maki 2010, 411; Johns 2011, 274).

82. **a, c** The designation of the principal diagnosis depends on the circumstances of the admission. In this case the patient has psychosis and this should be sequenced first with the substance coded second (Brown 2012, 143).

83. **c, d, e** Ventilator-associated pneumonia is assigned with the additional code for the organism. No other pneumonia code is assigned in additional to ventilator associated pneumonia (Brown 2012, 184).

84. **b, c, d, f** *Status asthmaticus* is defined as continual wheezing in spite of therapy (Brown 2012,186).

85. **a, c, e, f** Gastrointestinal bleeding manifests itself in several ways. These are hematemesis, melena, occult bleeding, hematochezia (Brown 2012, 201).

86. **c, e, f**   Codes for mechanical ventilation indicate whether the patient was on mechanical ventilation for fewer than 96 hours or more than 96 hours. The start time for calculating the duration begins with the start time of endotracheal tube insertion as the best method, followed by mechanical ventilation or the time that a patient who is on mechanical ventilation is admitted. The time ends with discontinuance of mechanical ventilation (Brown 2012, 194–195).

87. **a, c, d, f**   Both augmentation of breast for improved appearance and reduction of breast size are considered types of reconstruction (Brown 2012, 230).

88. **b, d, f**   The three types of pacemakers are single chamber, single chamber rate responsive, and dual chamber. A single chamber uses a single lead; a dual chamber requires two leads, one in the atrium and one in the ventricle. The leads should also be coded (Brown 2012, 358–359).

89. **d, e**   The open biopsy is performed prior to the definitive surgery so that the pathologist can perform a frozen section of the tissue to determine malignancy. Approaches, suturing, and closure are not coded separately. Exploratory surgery is not coded when definitive surgery is performed (Brown 2012, 68–71).

EXAM 2—PATIENT 1

PDX	836.1	Tear of lateral cartilage or meniscus of knee, current
DX2	844.2	Sprains and strains, cruciate ligament of knee
PP1	29881–RT	Arthroscopy, knee, surgical; with meniscectomy (medical OR lateral, including meniscal shaving)
PR2	29888–RT	Arthroscopically aided anterior cruciate ligament repair/augmentation or reconstruction

Notes on Outpatient 1

836.1   The condition requiring repair (Brown 2012, chapters 19 and 26).

844.2   An additional condition requiring surgery (Brown 2012, chapter 26).

29881–RT   Code is used for the repair of the meniscectomy (*CPT Assistant* Feb. 1996, 9; June 1999, 11; Aug. 2001, 7; Oct. 2003, 11; April 2005, 14; Dec. 2007, 10; *CPT Changes: An Insider's View* 2012).

29888–RT   Represents the arthroscopic repair of the ligament (*CPT Assistant* Oct. 2003, 11; Dec. 2007, 10).

EXAM 2—PATIENT 2

PDX	727.1	Bunion
PP1	28296–TA	Correction, hallux valgus (bunion), with or without sesamoidectomy; with metatarsal osteotomy (eg, Mitchell, Chevron, or concentric type procedures)

Notes on Outpatient 2

727.1   This is the code for a bunion and the definition for bunion can be found in *Dorland's Medical Dictionary* (Kuehn 2012, 127–128).

28296-TA   Third-party payers require submission of CPT codes with various modifiers, such as –TA for left foot, great toe (AMA *CPT Professional Edition* 2013, Modifier Section, inside front cover). This type of bunionectomy is described in the medical record (*CPT Assistant* Dec. 1996, 6; Jan. 2007, 31).

EXAM 2—PATIENT 3

PDX	493.92	Asthma with (acute) exacerbation
PP1	99284–25	E/M code based on mapping scenario provided
PR2	96365	Intravenous infusion, for therapy, prophylaxis, or diagnosis (specify substance or drug); initial, up to 1 hour

Notes on Outpatient 3

493.92   This condition brought the patient to the emergency department (Brown 2012, 186–187).

99284–25   This code represents the evaluation and management code for the facility APV and is done according to the mapping scenario as follows; meds given are = 2 = 5 points, the history is problem focused = 10 points, the exam is extended problem focused = 15 points, the number of tests = 4 = 15 points, supplies = one venipuncture set and one intravenous set = 10 points. 55 total points.

96365   The IV infusion is separately reportable and an additional code should be assigned (*CPT Changes: An Insider's View* 2009).

Note: The patient came to the ED because of asthma. The code that represents the most complicated process is the evaluation and management of the patient represented by the E/M code and is sequenced first. The starting of the IV is less complicated and sequenced second.

EXAM 2—PATIENT 4

PDX	789.01	Abdominal pain, right upper quadrant
DX2	787.01	Nausea with vomiting
DX3	276.51	Dehydration
DX4	530.81	Gastroesophageal reflux
DX5	300.00	Anxiety
PP1	99285–25	Evaluation and management mapping for case hospital visit level 5

Notes on Outpatient 4

789.01   This is the most severe symptom and the reason for the encounter (Brown 2012, 98).

787.01   This is a secondary condition that was evaluated and treated (Brown 2012, 98).

276.51   This is a secondary condition that was evaluated and treated (Brown 2012, 30).

530.81   This is a secondary condition that was evaluated and treated (Brown 2012, 203).

300.00   This is coded but does not fit within the requirements of four diagnoses required by the exam procedures.

99285–25   This is code is used to represent the evaluation and management code for the facility APV and is done according to the mapping scenario as follows; meds ordered are = 3 = 10 points, the history is comprehensive = 25 points, the exam is extended problem focused = 15 points, the number of tests = 6 = 20 points, supplies = 1 IV = 5 points. 75 total points.

EXAM 2—PATIENT 5

PDX	414.01	Coronary atherosclerosis of native coronary artery
PP1	92928-LD	Percutaneous transcatheter placement of intracoronary stent(s), with coronary angioplasty when performed; single major coronary artery or branch
PR2	93458	Left heart catheterization including intraprocedural injections for left ventriculography, imaging supervision and interpretation

Notes on Outpatient 5

414.01   This is the reason for the heart catheterization (Brown 2012, chapter 24).

92928   This code identifies the insertion of the drug-eluting stent into the left anterior descending coronary artery. The stenting procedure and is not reported separately because only the most complex procedure is coded (Kuehn 2012, 259–260).

–LD   The –LD modifier is used to identify that the PTCA/stent was completed in the left anterior descending coronary artery.

93458   This was a new code in 2011 for cardiac catheterization and angiography (*CPT Changes: An Insider's View* 2011, 186).

EXAM 2—PATIENT 6

PDX	338.3	Neoplasm related pain (acute) (chronic)
DX2	154.3	Malignant neoplasm, anus, unspecified
DX3	198.0	Secondary malignant neoplasm, kidney
DX4	197.0	Secondary malignant neoplasm, lung
DX5	198.3	Secondary malignant neoplasm, brain and spinal cord
DX6	401.9	Essential hypertension, unspecified
DX7	345.90	Epilepsy, unspecified (Seizure disorder NOS)
PP1	36569	Insertion of peripherally inserted central venous catheter (PICC), without subcutaneous port or pump; age 5 years or older
PR2	77001	Fluoroscopic guidance for central venous access device placement, replacement (catheter only or complete), or removal (includes fluoroscopic guidance for vascular access and catheter manipulation, any necessary contrast injections through access site or catheter with related venography radiologic supervision and interpretation, and radiographic documentation of final catheter position) (List separately in addition to code for primary procedures)

Notes on Outpatient 6

338.3   The reason for the patient encounter is to manage pain due to cancer. In this case code 338.3 should be assigned. The underlying neoplasm is reported as an additional diagnosis (Brown 2012, 163).

154.3,   The primary site of the cancer (anal) as well as all secondary sites are coded (Brown 2012,
198.0,   380–381).
197.0,
198.3

401.9,   These conditions are coded because they are chronic conditions (Brown 2012, 30).
345.90

36569   This is the code for insertion of PICC line in patient age = and older (*CPT Assistant* Oct. 2004, 14; Dec. 2004, 8; May 2005, 13; June 2008, 8).

77001   This is coded to represent the fluoroscopic guidance (*CPT Assistant* March 2007, 7; July 2008, 9).

EXAM 2—PATIENT 7

PDX	681.10	Cellulitis and abscess, toe
DX2	707.15	Ulcer of other part of foot
DX3	355.8	Mononeuritis of lower limb, unspecified
DX4	244.9	Unspecified hypothyroidism
DX5	401.9	Essential hypertension, unspecified
PP1	10060	Incision and drainage of abscess (eg, carbuncle, suppurative hidradenitis, cutaneous or subcutaneous abscess, cyst, furuncle, or paronychia); simple or single

Notes on Outpatient 7

681.10	The patient has an abscess/cellulitis of the toe (Brown 2012 242–243).
707.15	This condition is coded as it related to the abscess (Brown 2012, 242).
355.8	This condition is coded as it is a chronic condition (Brown 2012, 161).
244.9	This condition is coded as it is a chronic condition (Brown 2012, chapter 11).
401.9	This condition is coded as it is a chronic condition (Brown 2012, 346).
10060	(AMA *CPT Professional Edition* 2013, 63).

EXAM 2—PATIENT 8

PDX	656.41	Intrauterine death, delivered, with or without mention of antepartum condition
DX2	653.41	Fetopelvic disproportion, delivered, with or without mention of antepartum condition
DX3	663.31	Other and unspecified cord entanglement, without mention of compression, delivered, with or without mention of antepartum condition
DX4	649.11	Obesity complicating pregnancy, childbirth, or the puerperium, delivered, with or without mention of antepartum condition
DX5	278.00	Obesity, unspecified
DX6	V27.1	Single stillborn
PP1	74.0	Classical cesarean section
PR2	73.09	Other artificial rupture of membranes (not for induction of labor)
PR3	75.32	Fetal EKG (scalp)

Notes on Inpatient 8

663.31   Used to denote the nuchal cord without compression as documented in the operative report (Brown 2012, 281).

649.11   Obesity in pregnancy and delivery as documented in the history and physical (Brown 2012, chapter 20).

278.00   Coded to add further specificity to category 649.11 (Brown 2012, 129).

V27.1   Outcome of delivery for stillborn code (Brown 2012, 270).

73.09   Used to denote the artificial rupture of membranes performed after Pitocin is administered and labor fails to progress as documented in the H & P (Brown 2012, 282).

75.32   Use of internal fetal monitor (Brown 2012, 282).

Note: Per the Procedures for Coding Medical Record Cases for the CCS Examination (in the Introduction of this book), "Code all procedures that fall within the code range 00.01–86.99, but do not code 57.94 (Foley catheter)."

Points of Interest on Inpatient 8

1. This is an example of a very unfortunate situation of a baby's death. The intrauterine death is sequenced first because it is the reason for the cesarean section. Although it was thought the patient had cephalopelvic disproportion, the urgency of undertaking the cesarean section was due to the lack of fetal heart tones.

2. Code 73.4 is not assigned because it is not documented. In practice, the coder would query the physician.

EXAM 2—PATIENT 9

PDX	966.4	Accidental Poisoning of anti-Parkinsonism drugs
DX2	276.51	Dehydration
DX3	787.91	Diarrhea
DX4	E855.0	Accidental Poisoning, anti-Parkinsonism drugs
DX5	332.0	Paralysis agitans (Parkinsonism or Parkinson's disease)
DX6	530.81	Esophageal reflux
DX7	403.91	Hypertensive chronic kidney disease, unspecified
DX8	428.0	Congestive heart failure, unspecified
DX9	585.5	Chronic kidney disease, stage V

Notes on Inpatient 9

966.4   Poisoning due to Sinemet (Brown 2012, 445).

276.51   Dehydration is documented in the H & P and discharge summary and is the focus of treatment. Diarrhea and dehydration are both treated. Sequence 276.51 first because this condition is the focus of treatment (*Coding Clinic* 2nd Quarter 1988, 9; Brown 2012, 29).

787.91   Diarrhea (*Coding Clinic* 3rd Quarter 1995, 10; Brown 2012, 445).

E855.0   Poisoning of Sinemet (Brown 2012, 445).

332.0   Parkinson's disease is documented in the discharge summary (Brown 2012, 166).

530.81   Esophageal reflux is documented in the discharge summary (Brown 2012, 208–210).

428.0   Documented in the medical record and treated. Based on UHDDS criteria, the CHF is evaluated and monitored. Patient is also receiving medication, and CHF is a chronic condition. For all these reasons, this condition should be coded (Brown 2012, 339–340).

403.91,   Both are documented in the discharge summary. *ICD-9-CM Official Guidelines for Coding*

585.5   *and Reporting* (HHS 2011, Section I, C, 7, a) require both the combination hypertension code and chronic kidney disease code (Brown 2012, chapter 24).

Points of Interest on Inpatient 9

1. The crux of coding this case revolves around the poisoning from Sinemet. This is somewhat challenging because Sinemet is not in the *ICD-9-CM Official Guidelines for Coding and Reporting*. It is, however, a common anti-Parkinson's drug. An experienced coder should know this drug is associated with this disease and subsequently understand how to code a poisoning.

EXAM 2—PATIENT 10

PDX	287.31	Immune thrombocytopenic purpura (ITP)
DX2	571.2	Alcoholic cirrhosis of liver
DX3	250.01	Diabetes mellitus without mention of complication, type 1 [juvenile type], not stated as uncontrolled
DX4	303.93	Other and unspecified alcohol dependence, in remission
DX5	414.00	Coronary atherosclerosis of unspecified type of vessel, native or graft
DX6	518.52	Pulmonary insufficiency following trauma and surgery
DX7	272.4	Other and unspecified hyperlipidemia
DX8	401.9	Essential hypertension, unspecified
DX9	V45.81	Aortocoronary bypass status
DX10	V12.54	Personal history of transient ischemic attack (TIA), and cerebral infarction without residual deficits
PP1	41.5	Total splenectomy
PR2	96.71	Continuous invasive mechanical ventilation for less than 96 consecutive hours
PR3	96.04	Insertion of endotracheal tube

Notes on Inpatient 10

287.31   Idiopathic thrombocytopenic purpura is documented in the H & P and discharge summary (Brown 2012, chapter 13).

571.2,   Cirrhosis of the liver is diagnosed with this condition in association with the alcohol use in
303.93   the progress notes on 6/24. The fifth digit 3 was used because the patient stopped the alcohol one year before admission (Brown 2012, chapter 12).

250.01,   These chronic conditions should be coded as it meets the UHDDS criteria for an "other
414.00   diagnosis" (HHS 2011 Section III, 89).

518.52   Postoperative respiratory distress is documented in the 6/24 progress notes (Brown 2012, chapter 15).

272.4,   Chronic conditions that are being treated and therefore meet the UHDDS criteria as "other"
401.9   diagnoses.

V45.81   The history of these cardiovascular conditions likely contributes to the overall morbidity
V12.54 of this patient and must be considered as part of the patient's monitoring during the admission (Brown 2012, chapter 8).

41.5   Splenectomy documented on the operative report (Brown 2012, chapter 7).

96.04,   These conditions are coded as they are treating the postoperative respiratory distress based
96.71   on documentation on 6/24 (Brown 2012, 194).

Points of Interest on Inpatient 10

1. As is evident from the documentation, this case provides practice coding respiratory distress following surgery.

2. This case also provides the opportunity to code alcoholism and a related physical condition.

3. According to the Procedures for Coding Medical Record Cases for the CCS Examination (in the Introduction of this book), 99.05 transfusion platelet and 99.04 transfusion of PRBC are not coded as per exam specifications.

EXAM 2—PATIENT 11

PDX	428.0	Congestive heart failure, unspecified
DX2	397.0	Diseases of tricuspid valve
DX3	250.01	Diabetes mellitus without mention of complication, type 1 [juvenile type], not stated as uncontrolled
DX4	110.1	Dermatophytosis of nail
DX5	703.8	Diseases of nail, hypertrophy
DX6	401.9	Essential hypertension, unspecified
DX7	305.1	Tobacco use disorder
PP1	86.27	Debridement of nail, nail bed, or nail fold
PR2	86.27	Debridement of nail, nail bed, or nail fold

Notes on Inpatient 11

428.0   The patient is admitted with CHF as documented on the H & P and discharge summary. Even though the patient also has tricuspid valve insufficiency, use the 428.0 because, there is no documentation the CHF is rheumatic (*Coding Clinic* 2nd Quarter 2000, 16–17; Brown 2012, 339–340).

397.0   Tricuspid insufficiency is documented on the discharge summary and H & P (Brown 2012, 330–331).

250.01   Diabetes mellitus type 1 is documented on the discharge summary and H & P. The V code is not used because type 1 diabetes requires insulin (Brown 2012, 121–123; *Coding Clinic* 4th Quarter 2004, 55).

110.1   Mycotic nails (703.8), Hypertrophic nails (401.9), Hypertension (305.1), and tobacco abuse are all documented in the medical record and meet the UHDDS definition (HHS, 2011, Section III, 89). 305.1 does not require a fifth digit (HHS 2011, Tabular Index).

86.27   Debridement of nails performed as per the progress notes and the consult sheet. As per the Procedures for Coding Medical Record Cases for the CCS Examination (in the Introduction of this book), "Code all procedures that fall within the code range 00.01–86.99, but do not code 57.94 (Foley catheter)." This is coded twice because it is a bilateral debridement.

Points of Interest on Inpatient 11

1. This case provides an example of the coding rules for coding congestive heart failure with a heart valve disorder (*Coding Clinic* 2nd Quarter 2000, 16–17).

2. The documentation is interesting because the only place the procedure is documented is in the consultation. This is a practice in some healthcare facilities and illustrates the need to review every document in the record in order to code accurately.

EXAM 2—PATIENT 12

PDX	634.11	Spontaneous abortion complicated by delayed or excessive hemorrhage, incomplete
DX2	649.03	Tobacco use disorder complicating pregnancy, childbirth, or the puerperium, antepartum condition or complication
DX3	648.43	Other current conditions in the mother complicating pregnancy, mental disorders, antepartum complication
DX4	311	Depressive disorder, not elsewhere classified
DX5	305.01	Alcohol abuse, continuous
PP1	69.02	Dilatation and curettage following delivery or abortion

Notes on Inpatient 12

634.11 — This is a case of an incomplete spontaneous abortion. This is evidenced by the pathology report. The patient has documented heavy bleeding that has resulted in anemia. Therefore, use the fourth digit 1 and a fifth digit 1 (Brown 2012, 278–279).

649.03 — Tobacco abuse is also documented and treated. The pregnancy (649.03) code is specific to tobacco abuse and because of this, only use one code (Brown 2012, 277, 296).

69.02 — The patient underwent a D & C following spontaneous abortion (Brown 2012, 294).

648.43, 311, 305.01 — These conditions are coded to add further specificity. Alcohol abuse is treated and relevant to the case. The physician documented the patient had "alcohol abuse," even though clinically the patient may have alcoholism. Therefore, alcohol abuse, the diagnosis that is documented, is the one that is coded (*Coding Clinic* 2nd Quarter 1998, 13–14). The fifth digit 3 is used as the patient did not deliver and the conditions were antepartum (Brown 2012, 277).

Points of Interest on Inpatient 12

1. This case illustrates the difference between coding an incomplete spontaneous abortion and a complication of abortion. In the documentation of the record, the patient had a D & C to complete the spontaneous abortion. A coder might think this should be coded with a code from the 639 category. However, if there are products of conception or other material from the pregnancy retained in the uterus at the time of readmission, this indicates the abortion was not completed. Therefore, use the 634 category. If, on the other hand, there was no retained material, use the 639 category (complication of spontaneous abortion).

2. Spontaneous abortion and miscarriage are used interchangeably in *ICD-9-CM Official Guidelines for Coding and Reporting*.

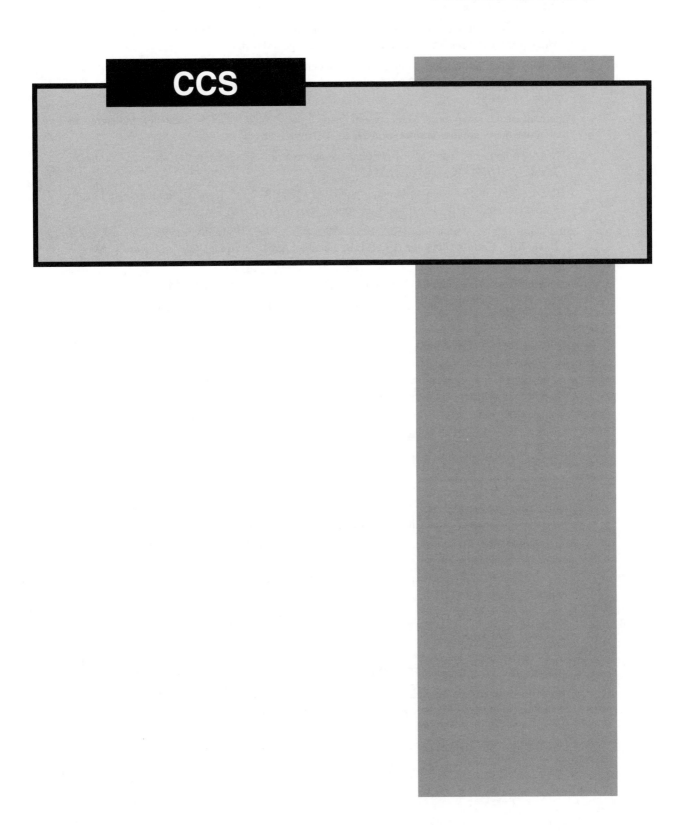

References

CCS

References

American College of Radiology (ACR) and the Radiological Society of North America (RSNA). 2010 (March). CT Colonography: http://www.radiologyinfo.org/en/info.cfm?pg=ct_colo.

American Health Information Management Association. 2012. *Pocket Glossary of Health Information Management and Technology*, Third Edition. Chicago: AHIMA.

American Health Information Management Association. 2011 (Oct. 2). Code of Ethics. http://library .ahima.org/xpedio/groups/public/documents/ahima/bok1_024277.hcsp?dDocName=bok1_024277. Chicago: AHIMA.

American Health Information Management Association. 2008 (Oct.). Practice Brief: Managing an effective query process. *Journal of AHIMA* 79(10): 83–88.

AHIMA Compliance Task Force. 1999 (Jan.). Practice Brief: Seven Steps to Corporate Compliance. *Journal of AHIMA*. Chicago: AHIMA.

AHIMA e-HIM Work Group on Maintaining the Legal EHR. 2005. Update: Maintaining a Legally Sound Health Record—Paper and Electronic. *Journal of AHIMA* 76(10): 64A–L.

American Hospital Association. 1984, 1987–1990, 1992, 1993, 1995, 1997, 1998, 2000, 2001, 2002, 2004–2011. *Coding Clinic for ICD-9-CM*. Chicago: AHA Services. *(Refer to the answer key for specifics.)*

American Medical Association. 2013. *CPT Professional Edition*. Chicago: AMA.

American Medical Association. 2006, 2009, 2010, 2011, 2012. *CPT Changes Insider's View*. Chicago: AMA. *(Refer to the answer key for specifics.)*

American Medical Association. 1995, 1996, 1999, 2000, 2001, 2003, 2005, 2008, 2009, 2010, 2011, 2012. *CPT Assistant*. Chicago: AMA. *(Refer to the answer key for specifics.)*

America Pregnancy Association (APA). 2007. Cephalopelvic disproportion (CPD): www.americanpregnancy.org/labornbirth/cephalopelvicdisproportion.html.

Bowman, Sue. 2007. *Health Information Management Compliance Guidelines for Preventing Fraud and Abuse*, Fourth Edition. Chicago: AHIMA.

Brodnik, Melanie, McCain, Mary, Rinehart-Thompson, Laurie, and Rebecca Reynolds. 2009. *Fundamentals of Law for Health Informatics and Health Information Management*. Chicago: AHIMA.

Brown, Faye (author) and Nelly Leon-Chisen (editor). 2012. *ICD-9-CM Coding Handbook with Answers*, Revised Edition. Chicago: AHA Services.

Casto, Anne B. and Elizabeth Layman. 2011. *Principles of Healthcare Reimbursement, Third Edition*. Chicago: AHIMA.

Clark, Andrea. 2009 (March). "Key Issues in the 2009 OPPS Final Rule" *Journal of AHIMA* 80(3):72–73.

Centers for Medicare and Medicaid Services (CMS). 2012. https://www.cms.gov/ QualityImprovementOrgs

Centers for Medicare and Medicaid Services (CMS). 2011. https://www.cms.gov/acuteinpatientpps/ ipps2011/itemdetail.asp?itemid=CMS1237948

Center for Medicare and Medicaid (CMS) Division of Institutional Claims Processing. 2008. "Definition and Uses of Health Insurance Prospective Payment System Codes (HIPPS Codes). https://www.cms .gov/ProspMedicareFeeSvcPmtGen/downloads/hippsusesv4.pdf.

Davis, Nadinia and Melissa LaCour. 2007. *Health Information Technology*. Philadelphia: Saunders.

DeVault, Kathy. 2010. CPT Coding Updates. *Journal of AHIMA* 81(2):62–63, 66. Chicago: AHIMA.

Dorland's Medical Dictionary, 27ᵗʰ ed. 2000. Baltimore: Lippincott, Williams and Wilkins.

Garrett, Gail S. 2009. *Present on Admission*, Second Edition. Chicago: AHIMA.

Hazelwood, Anita C., and Carol A. Venable. 2011. *ICD-9-CM Diagnostic Coding and Reimbursement for Physician Services.* Chicago: AHIMA.

Johns, Merida (volume editor). 2011. *Health Information Management Technology*, Third Edition. Chicago: AHIMA.

Kuehn, Lynn. 2012. *Procedural Coding and Reimbursement for Physician Services: Applying Current Procedural Terminology and HCPCS.* Chicago: AHIMA.

LaTour, Kathleen and Shirley Eichenwald Maki (volume editors) 2010. *Health Information Management: Concepts, Principles, and Practice*, Third Edition. Chicago: AHIMA.

Lovaasen, K.R. and Schwerdtfeger, J. 2011. *ICD-9-CM Coding: Theory and Practice*, 2ⁿᵈ Edition. Health Sciences Division: Elsevier.

McWay, D. C. 2003. *Legal Aspects of health Information Management*, 2ⁿᵈ Edition. Delmar Cengage Learning.

Medicare Grouper. 2011. Version 29-10/11.

Schraffenberger, Lou Ann. 2012. *Basic ICD-10-CM/PCS and ICD-9-CM Coding.* Chicago: AHIMA.

Schraffenberger, Lou Ann and Kuehn, Lynn. 2011. *Effective Management of Coding Services.* Chicago: AHIMA.

Scott, Karen S. 2009. *Coding and Reimbursement for Hospital Inpatient Services*, 2ⁿᵈ Edition. Chicago: AHIMA.

Smith, Gail I. 2013. *Basic Current Procedural Terminology and HCPCS Coding*, 2013. Chicago: AHIMA.

US Department of Health and Human Services (HHS). 2011. International Classification of Diseases, Ninth Revision, Clinical Modification (ICD-9-CM). http://www.cdc.gov/nchs/icd/icd9cm.htm.

US Department of Health and Human Services. 2003 (Jan. 1). Medicare Conditions of Participation: Medical Staff: http://www.access.gpo.gov/nara/cfr/waisidx_03/42cfr482_03.html.

Additional Resources

AHIMA Communities of Practice (CoP): http://cop.ahima.org

AHIMA Certification: www.ahima.org/certification

ICD-9-CM Coding

Clinical Coding Workout: Practice Exercises for Skill Development (with Answers). 2012. Chicago: AHIMA.

HCPCS and CPT Coding

Principles of CPT Coding. Chicago: American Medical Association.

http://www.cms.gov/HCPCSReleaseCodeSets/ANHCPCS/list.asp#TopOfPage (Search for FY 11) 2011_CCS_References.docx

Regulatory Guidelines, Data Quality, and Compliance

Books

Kennedy, James S. 2008. *Severity DRGs and Reimbursement:* An MS-DRG Primer. Chicago: AHIMA.

2011 DRG Desk Reference. 2011. Ingenix.

Websites

APCs and status indicators (for 2011): https://www.cms.gov/HospitalOutpatientPPS/ (Search for *addendum B.*)

Common medications and associated diseases: www.rxlist.com

Decision trees, stress management, and other topics: http://www.mindtools.com/dectree.html. *(Note: Decision trees form the basis of DRG trees, which are found on the national exam. It is important to review this Web site.)*

DRG grouper (free): irp.com *(Disclaimer: This software application may contain errors and is not endorsed or developed by the author or AHIMA.)*

MS-DRG weights for 2011: https://www.cms.gov/AcuteInpatientPPS/FFD/list.asp#TopOfPage (Search for FY 2011 DRG weights.)

Present on admission information: http://www.cms.hhs.gov/HospitalAcqCond/01_Overview.asp

Documentation, Information and Communication Technologies and Privacy, Confidentiality, Legal, and Ethical Issues

Thomason, Mary C. 2008. *HIPAA by Example*. Chicago: AHIMA.

Amatayakul, Margret K. 2009. *Electronic Health Records: A Practical Guide for Professionals and Organizations*, Fourth Edition. Chicago: AHIMA.